D0940758

How the ENDOCRINE SYSTEM *Works*

About the Cover

The cover features a photographic image of the cross-section of an ovary containing struma ovarii, a rare condition in which ectopic thyroid tissue is present in the ovary. This image is used with the permission of Dr. Peter A. Kubiczek, Department of Pathology, Ball Memorial Hospital, Muncie, IN.

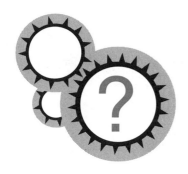

How the
ENDOCRINE SYSTEM
Works

By

J. MATTHEW NEAL, MD, FACP, FACE

Director, Internal Medicine Residency
Ball Memorial Hospital
Muncie, Indiana

Clinical Associate Professor of Medicine
Indiana University School of Medicine
Muncie Center for Medical Education
Muncie, Indiana

Series Editor

LAUREN SOMPAYRAC, PhD

b

**Blackwell
Science**

©2001 by Blackwell Science, Inc.

Editorial Offices:
Commerce Place, 350 Main Street, Malden, Massachusetts 02148, USA
Osney Mead, Oxford OX2 0EL, England
25 John Street, London WC1N 2BL, England
23 Ainslie Place, Edinburgh EH3 6AJ, Scotland
54 University Street, Carlton, Victoria 3053, Australia

Other Editorial Offices:
Blackwell Wissenschafts-Verlag GmbH, Kurfürstendamm 57, 10707 Berlin, Germany
Blackwell Science KK, MG Kodenmacho Building, 7-10 Kodenmacho Nihombashi, Chuo-ku, Tokyo 104, Japan
Iowa State University Press, A Blackwell Science Company, 2121 S. State Avenue, Ames, Iowa 50014-8300, USA

Distributors:

USA
Blackwell Science, Inc.
Commerce Place
350 Main Street
Malden, Massachusetts 02148
(Telephone orders: 800-215-1000 or 781-388-8250; fax orders: 781-388-8270)

Canada
Login Brothers Book Company
324 Saulteaux Crescent
Winnipeg, Manitoba R3J 3T2
(Telephone orders: 204-837-2987)

Australia
Blackwell Science Pty, Ltd.
54 University Street
Carlton, Victoria 3053
(Telephone orders: 03-9347-0300;
fax orders: 03-9349-3016)

Outside North America and Australia
Blackwell Science, Ltd.
c/o Marston Book Services, Ltd.
P.O. Box 269
Abingdon
Oxon OX14 4YN
England
(Telephone orders: 44-01235-465500;
fax orders: 44-01235-465555)

All rights reserved. No part of this book may be reproduced in any form or by any electronic or mechanical means, including information storage and retrieval systems, without permission in writing from the publisher, except by a reviewer who may quote brief passages in a review.

Acquisitions: Nancy Anastasi Duffy
Development: Nancy Anastasi Duffy
Production: Shawn Girsberger
Manufacturing: Lisa Flanagan
Marketing Manager: Toni Fournier
Cover design by Meral Dabcovich, Visual Perspectives
Interior design by Diane Lorenz, Lorenz Computer Graphics, Boulder, CO
Typeset by Software Services
Printed and bound by Edwards Brothers / Ann Arbor

Printed in the United States of America
01 02 03 04 5 4 3 2 1

The Blackwell Science logo is a trade mark of Blackwell Science Ltd., registered at the United Kingdom Trade Marks Registry

Library of Congress Cataloging-in-Publication Data

Neal, J. Matthew.
  How the endocrine system works / J. Matthew Neal.
    p. ; cm.
Includes index.
  ISBN 0-632-04556-6 (pbk.)
  1. Endocrine glands—Physiology. 2. Endocrine glands—Diseases. 3. Hormones—Physiological effect.
  [DNLM: 1. Endocrine System—physiology. 2. Endocrine Diseases. WK 102 N341h 2001] I. Title.
  QP187 .N35 2001
  612.4—dc21
                                                                    2001001141

I am grateful to many individuals who assisted me during the development of this book. I would like to thank my editor at Blackwell Science, Chris Davis, who asked me to write this book and was very helpful during the development process. I am also very grateful to Dr. Lauren Sompayrac, the editor of this series, who provided much feedback during the writing process. I thank Shawn Girsberger, at Blackwell Science, who helped me tremendously in creating suitable graphic art files. I could not have completed this project without my nurse Emily Daugherty who took care of many messages in the office and shielded me from intruders during the many hours of dedicated writing time that was necessary. I thank my endocrinology partners Dr. Kurt Alexander and Dr. Clark Perry, who were always available to provide advice and criticism when necessary. I would like to thank many of my residents and medical students who offered helpful advice. And finally, I would like to thank my wife Alexis who was extremely helpful and patient during this project.

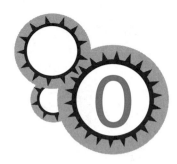

HOW TO USE THIS BOOK

I wrote this book as an overview of the endocrine system. It is not intended for endocrinologists, but instead for those desiring a succinct introduction to this fascinating branch of medicine. It is not meant to be a comprehensive text or examination study guide, as many such books are readily available. I wanted something that you could sit down with and readily assimilate in a few evenings.

How the Endocrine System Works is written in a lecture format, as if I were talking to you personally. It is designed to be read from start to finish, and to be as entertaining as possible. (Some would dispute that endocrinology could ever be entertaining!) I have tried to interject some humor into the subject matter, and from time to time mention interesting historical events in endocrinology, such as the discovery of insulin and cortisone. I have stressed the basics while avoiding excessive detail—as well as excessive simplicity.

This book may be used alone in an introductory course, or as a companion to a more detailed textbook. However you are using it, I hope that you enjoy it! Please feel free to provide any feedback to me regarding this text.

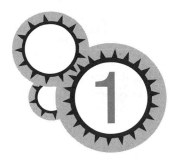

AN OVERVIEW

Endocrinology is the study of endocrine glands and their secretions. It can be a difficult topic to master because of all the mechanisms and feedback loops to understand. One way to understand the endocrine system is to break it down into smaller parts, and that is what I have attempted to accomplish in this book. It may help to visualize each endocrine system as part of a much larger group; envision a football team with all the players (quarterback, running backs, center, guards, receivers, punter, etc.). Each of these players must perform his job properly for the team to win. If even one player is out of sync, the play may be botched. The quarterback is in charge of the team, calls the plays, and provides leadership.

Football teams often communicate plays with audible signals. Organisms also require communication; they have developed hormones to send messages or commands from one part of the organism to another. Simple, one-celled organisms did not have a great need for complex endocrine systems. But as organisms became more complex, large intercellular communication mechanisms became necessary for homeostasis. The word "hormone" is derived from the Greek word meaning "arouse to activity." To many lay people, the word "hormone" conjures up images of estrogen or thyroid replacement therapy. In fact, there are many types of hormones, with new ones discovered every day. The endocrine system sends signals to the body by secreting hormones (e.g., insulin, growth hormone, thyroxine) directly into the circulation. In contrast, the exocrine glands secrete their substances into a duct system (e.g., sweat glands, exocrine pancreas).

The endocrine system is composed of many different glands throughout the body. The endocrine glands may be divided into two categories. The first, or "classical" glands' function is primarily endocrine in nature. The second, or "nonclassical" glands' primary function is something else but they also secrete important substances.

The "classical" endocrine glands include the anterior pituitary, thyroid, parathyroids, adrenal cortex and medulla, gonads (testes and ovaries), and the endocrine pancreas. The primary function of these glands is to manufacture specific hormones. Some nonclassical endocrine organs and their hormones include the heart (atrial natriuretic peptide), brain (hypothalamic hormones), kidney (calcitriol, renin), liver (IGF-I, angiotensin II), lymphocytes (cytokines, interleukins), GI tract (gastrin, secretin, vasoactive intestinal peptide), and many others. Many of the "classical" hormones are under the control of the hypothalamus and pituitary, which may be thought of as extensions of the nervous system. Indeed, the nervous and endocrine systems may function together quite closely (neuroendocrinology).

FUNCTION OF HORMONES

So why are hormones so important, anyway? The first thing that an organism must have in order to survive is energy. Food must be converted into energy, excess energy needs to be converted to storage, and stored energy must be mobilized when necessary to meet the organism's needs. In the chapter on glucose metabolism, we will learn the effects of insulin and glucagon on the body's metabolism. Thyroid hormones are important in regulation of the body's metabolism. Glycogen and lipids are necessary to provide long-term energy needs when food is not available.

The organism must maintain its internal environment. Many hormones play a role here. Hormones such as antidiuretic hormone, aldosterone, and atrial natriuretic peptide are important in water and sodium balance. Calcium is necessary for many bodily functions, and its metabolism is regulated by parathyroid hormone, calcitonin, and vitamin D. Several hormones, including thyroid hormones, growth hormone, and sex steroids, control growth and development.

And, finally, reproduction is essential for the continued survival of any organism. Specialized reproductive organs (gonads) produce sex steroids that are necessary for spermatogenesis and ovulation. Gonads are under the complex control of the hypothalamic-pituitary axis (HPA).

COMPOSITION OF HORMONES

Hormones are made from a variety of different molecules. The majority of hormones are of the protein or peptide variety. Proteins are chains of amino acids linked together. Some of these peptide hormones are only a few amino acids in length; most are much larger, with some being over 200 amino acids in length. Even the very small protein vasopressin (a nonapeptide) looks quite complex:

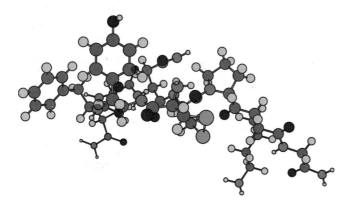

Glycoproteins are sort of a hybrid hormone, consisting of a peptide hormone associated with a carbohydrate moiety. Examples include LH (luteinizing hormone), FSH (follicle-stimulating hormone), TSH (thyroid-stimulating hormone or thyrotropin), and human chorionic gonadotropin (β-hCG). These hormones all share a common alpha subunit (α-SU); the beta subunits differ from one to another.

Instead of being linked together to form proteins, one or two amino acids may be modified to form hormones. The amino acid tyrosine is modified to form the catecholamines (e.g., epinephrine and norepinephrine). These hormones are very important in the nervous system. The thyroid or iodothyronine hormones (thyroxine, triiodothyronine) are made by joining two modified tyrosine molecules and adding several iodine atoms.

Tyrosine

Cholesterol, a molecule that we associate with atherosclerosis, is in fact essential to life. It is the precursor of steroid hormones—such as cortisol, aldosterone, estradiol, and testosterone—and sterol hormones, such as calcitriol.

Cholesterol

Another common hormone precursor is the fatty acid (the major storage component of fat), which serves as a precursor of hormones called eicosanoids. The most important eicosanoids, the prostaglandins, are derived from arachidonic acid. Other eicosanoids include thromboxanes, leukotrienes, and prostacyclins. They are important in smooth muscle contraction, hemostasis, inflammatory and immunologic responses, circulation, respiratory, and gastrointestinal systems.

Simple ions such as calcium also have hormone-like effects, and calcium metabolism will be discussed in Lecture 6.

HOW HORMONES WORK

Hormones must have a way to tell the other cells what to do. The end effect of a hormone is usually at the nucleus, resulting in production of a protein that has some effect on the cell. Some hormones go directly to the nucleus and have an effect there. These types of hormones tend to be ones that can easily traverse the cell membrane; for this to happen, the hormone usually must be "non-polar" (non-charged). These include the steroid and iodothyronine hormones.

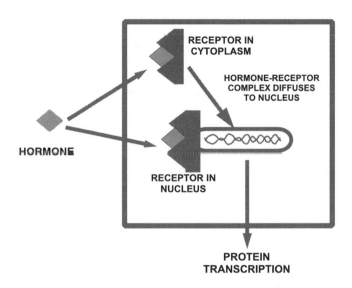

The second class of hormones has no direct effect but instead binds to cell surface receptors, which initiate production of one or more second messengers that carry out the action. One messenger may trigger another messenger, which may trigger yet another messenger, and so on. This concept of "multiple messengers" is called an amplification cascade and is the reason that some of these hormones are effective at extremely low concentrations (e.g., 10^{-12} moles per liter). An analogy to the game of football would be a running back carrying the ball behind his blockers. Without the blockers, he is likely to be tackled quite quickly; with multiple blockers, his power is "amplified" to the extent that many more yards can be gained before he is tackled. These hormones tend to be highly electrically charged, and include peptide, glycoprotein, and catecholamine hormones, and therefore cannot easily traverse the cell membrane.

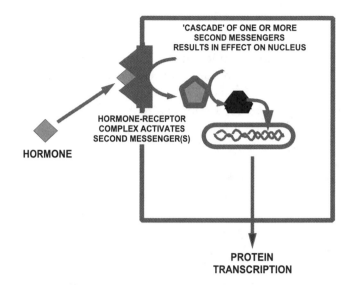

Another important difference between these hormones is how they travel in the blood. Those that act on the nucleus directly (e.g., steroids) tend to travel bound to a carrier protein. These carrier proteins may be specific for those hormones (e.g., sex-hormone binding globulin), or may be common proteins (e.g., albumin). The hormones are more slowly degraded if they are bound to carrier proteins.

The portion bound to the carrier protein is typically inactive. There is a small portion of the hormone that is not bound to the carrier protein and this is called the active or free portion. This is clinically significant because some common conditions may result in an increase or decrease in the amount of carrier protein. This does not affect the free (active) portion, but does affect the total amount of hormone present (free + bound). Many laboratories measure the total, not the free hormone level. Consequently, when there is a carrier protein abnormality, the total hormone may not accurately reflect the free level, which could lead to errors in diagnosis and management. Fortunately, many hormones can be measured in their free (unbound) state, which avoids this type of problem.

Peptide, glycoprotein, and catecholamine hormones are not bound to carrier proteins and thus the type of problem mentioned above does not apply. Because they travel unbound in the plasma, they are usually degraded more quickly than the carrier-protein hormones. Glycoproteins, because of their large carbohydrate component, are more slowly metabolized than pure peptide hormones.

HORMONAL REGULATION

Although endocrinology is very complex, much of it can be figured out if you understand the mechanisms. Most hormones have another hormone that regulates its secretion; a hormone that stimulates another hormone's secretion is called a trophic or stimulatory hormone. Those that cause less of the hormone to be secreted are called inhibitory hormones. The hormone thus secreted by the gland of interest causes a desired effect at the target gland's nucleus (e.g., production of a protein). Once this substance reaches a desired level, it tells the trophic hormone cells to slow down and stop stimulating the endocrine organ. This causes reduction in the hormone levels by a process called feedback inhibition. This keeps the whole system in check by preventing too much hormone from being synthesized. In effect, the end product of the endocrine organ becomes a type of indirect inhibitory hormone (by decreasing production of the trophic hormone).

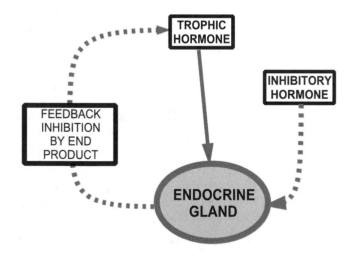

You may compare the concept of feedback inhibition to filling up your car with gas. You go to the gas station when your gauge says that the tank is empty. Problems may arise when the gauge malfunctions (e.g., you have a full tank when it reads empty, or vice versa). When you fill up the tank, the pump should stop delivering gas when the tank is full. If it stops too soon, the tank will not be full; if it does not stop after the tank is full, gas spills out all over the place. The purpose of feedback inhibition is to keep the "gas tank" at the correct level.

When something disrupts the normal feedback mechanisms, the endocrine system goes awry and hormonal abnormalities result. Let's think of some things that can go awry with the feedback mechanisms and cause disruption of the endocrine system:

1. Target organ is damaged or absent and produces insufficient hormone (hypofunction); it does not respond to trophic hormone stimulation (primary deficiency, e.g., hypothyroidism due to Hashimoto's thyroiditis or thyroidectomy).
2. Target organ produces too much hormone (hyperfunction); autonomous secretion of hormone occurs despite suppressed trophic hormone (e.g., Cushing's syndrome [cortisol hypersecretion] due to autonomously functioning adrenal tumor; hyperthyroidism due to toxic nodular goiter).
3. Receptor defect/hormone resistance: desired effect not produced despite large amounts of hormone (e.g., type 2 diabetes mellitus).
4. Excess trophic hormone that secondarily produces excess target organ hormone (e.g., Cushing's syndrome due to excess corticotropin [ACTH] production).
5. Deficiency of trophic hormone; inadequate target organ hormone produced despite structurally intact primary organ (secondary deficiency, e.g., hypopituitarism).
6. Administration of excess exogenous hormone (e.g., Cushing's syndrome due to excess corticosteroid administration).

INTERACTIONS BETWEEN THE ENDOCRINE AND IMMUNE SYSTEMS

It was recognized long ago that alterations in the immune system occur after significant change in the endocrine milieu (e.g., gonadectomy, pregnancy). This led to the proposition that there is an interaction between the immune and endocrine systems. Cytokines are extremely potent molecules secreted by immune cells that have significant regulatory effects on the endocrine system; in a way, they act as hormones themselves. At least 100 different cytokines have been isolated, and include the interleukins, tumor necrosis factors, interferons, transforming growth factors, and colony-stimulating factors. Such immune factors may either inhibit or potentiate endocrine secretion. For example, it was observed long ago that severe burn victims increased their corticosteroid and catecholamine production dramatically. Much of this increase can be explained by the effects of various inflammatory factors on the adrenal cortex and medulla. A very common condition called the euthyroid sick syndrome appears to be at least partially mediated by inflammatory products such as cytokines. A full discussion of this topic is extremely complex and beyond the scope of this text.

HORMONE MEASUREMENTS

Although we can measure most known hormones in the blood, the circumstances under which we measure them are very important. Random hormone levels are often of little use because many hormones are secreted in periodic or cyclical fashion, with levels varying throughout the day. For example, cortisol levels are typically highest in the morning, but lower in the evening. These levels would be the opposite in a person who works the "night shift" (i.e., works at night and sleeps during the day). Blind individuals sometimes lose this cyclical variation, so it appears that the presence of daylight may have some influence on this phenomenon.

To adequately study secretion of some hormones, we must perform a perturbation study in which a substance is given to produce a desired result (i.e., stimulation or inhibition of the hormone's secretion). If concerned about hormone deficiency, a stimulatory test is done by administering a secretagogue (substance that provokes a hormonal response). The hormone of interest is usually measured before, and at one or more intervals after, administration of the secretagogue.

If hormonal excess is suspected, then a suppression or inhibitory test is performed: a substance known to suppress hormone levels is administered. For example, random growth hormone (GH) levels are often not useful in evaluating GH excess (gigantism or acromegaly) because of the episodic secretion of pituitary hormones. Since hyperglycemia is a known inhibitor of GH secretion, a glucose suppression test is possible, in which GH levels are measured before and after a large oral glucose load. In normal health, GH is suppressed; in acromegaly, secretion is autonomous and it is not suppressed.

An alternative to a provocative test may be urine collection over a long period of time (e.g., 24 hours), which eliminates some of the problems associated with random hormone measurements. For example,

pheochromocytomas often secrete catecholamines intermittently, making random measurements useless. A 24-hour urine collection for catecholamines and metabolites will usually be elevated in these persons.

One must often use caution in the interpretation of "normal values" of laboratory tests. Most human measurements (height, weight, intelligence, etc.) and measurements of hormone function follow the normal distribution or "bell curve":

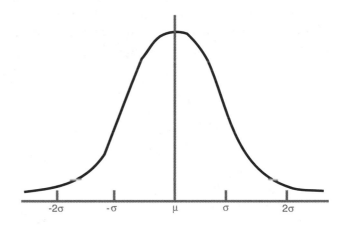

The normal distribution curve is symmetrical about the mean (μ) or 50th percentile. One and two standard deviations (σ) above the mean correspond approximately to the 84th and 97.5th percentiles, respectively; one and two standard deviations below the mean correspond to the 16th and 2.5th percentiles, respectively. A laboratory often defines "normal ranges" as a 95% confidence interval (two standard deviations above and below the mean); this means that by definition, 5% of "normal" persons fall outside the "normal range," and that minimally abnormal values may simply represent a normal variant.

In addition, "normal ranges" for some hormones may be quite large (e.g., the normal range for serum total thyroxine is approximately 5.0–12.0 µg/dL). So, it is possible for a person to have hypothyroidism with a "normal" T4 of 5.2 µg/dL; his or her "normal" might be 9 µg/dL. It is often useful, then, to measure both the hormone of interest and the trophic hormone (a "hormone pair"). Indeed, many patients with low normal-T4 levels have elevated TSH levels, indicating primary hypothyroidism. Measuring the pair often yields more information than either hormone measurement gives alone.

NOMENCLATURE OF ENDOCRINE DISORDERS

A normal endocrine state is denoted by the prefix "eu" (e.g., euglycemia, euthyroid, eucalcemic). Hypofunctional states contain the prefix "hypo" (e.g., hypoparathyroidism, hypopituitarism). Examples of hyperfunctional states include hyperthyroidism, hyperparathyroidism, and hyperinsulinism. These disorders may be classified more specifically. For example, there are many causes of hyperthyroidism, including Graves' disease, toxic nodular goiter, and subacute thyroiditis. Patients with elevated glucose levels are usually said to have diabetes mellitus rather than hyperglycemia.

HYPOFUNCTION

HORMONE DEFICIENCY SYNDROMES

Endocrine deficiency occurs if the primary (target) organ functions inadequately; this is a primary deficiency disorder. Examples include hypothyroidism due to Hashimoto's thyroiditis, Addison's disease (primary adrenal insufficiency), and type 1 diabetes mellitus. In primary disorders, the organ's trophic hormone level is elevated; for example, those with primary hypothyroidism have an elevated serum TSH level. The trophic hormone in this case is "beating a dead horse"—the gland does not work properly despite massive attempts to stimulate it.

Secondary deficiency disorders occur when the trophic hormone for the target organ is deficient. This occurs in hypopituitarism, in which the target organs (thyroid, adrenal, gonads) are structurally intact, but are not stimulated properly. Tertiary disorders are similar to secondary syndromes except that the deficiency is one step higher; i.e., the trophic hormone for the trophic gland is deficient. An example is hypothalamic dysfunction, in which the hypothalamic hormones are made in insufficient amounts to stimulate the pituitary, and in turn, the target organs.

Antibody-mediated (autoimmune) endocrine organ destruction is the most common cause of hormone deficiency. Our bodies normally produce antibodies to defend against invaders such as viruses and bacteria. Occasionally, however, the body may produce antibodies that attack its own organs, causing destruction. Inflammatory or infiltrative disease may also result in organ destruction and hormone deficiency. Patients with inflammation of the pancreas (pancreatitis) may develop diabetes due to insufficient insulin secretion. Hemochromatosis is a relatively common disorder of iron overload in which excessive iron deposits cause organ dysfunction. This disorder may cause diabetes and adrenal insufficiency.

Large tumors in or about the target organ may destroy enough cells to cause hormone deficiency. A common example is pituitary hormone deficiency (hypopituitarism), which is often caused by the destructive effects of large pituitary tumors.

HORMONE RESISTANCE

It is also possible for a hormone to be made in sufficient quantity but to have inadequate effect because of resistance to the hormone. Here, the patient's hormone receptors are either absent or insufficiently sensitive to the hormone for the desired effect to occur. This appears as a true endocrine deficiency disorder although normal or even increased amounts of the hormone are made. The most common example is type 2 diabetes mellitus, in which patients are insulin resistant. These patients develop elevated blood glucose levels (hyperglycemia). Very large amounts of exogenous insulin may be required to overcome the insulin resistance.

TREATMENT OF HORMONE DEFICIENCY

Ideally, we treat deficiency syndromes by replacing the native hormone, producing normal physiologic levels. This is pretty easy for orally absorbed molecules that have a relatively long half-life (e.g., thyroxine, hydrocortisone, estradiol). Some hormones, however, are not well absorbed orally. These include most peptide hormones, which are degraded in the gastrointestinal tract. Many of these are given by injection; examples include insulin and growth hormone. Some peptides are synthetically modified to have a longer duration in the blood; these include desmopressin (a derivative of vasopressin) and octreotide (an analog of somatostatin). Other hormones such as testosterone are absorbed orally, but are metabolized in the liver to inactive products (the first-pass phenomenon) before they get to the circulation.

These hormones also must be given by injection or transdermal (patch) preparation.

And, even if we have the hormone to provide, it may not be possible to replace it in a precise physiological fashion. The best example of this is type 1 diabetes mellitus, in which the patient is dependent on insulin injections to sustain life. It is impossible to mimic insulin secretion perfectly. At best, the patient must learn to live with compromises, such as occasional hyperglycemia and hypoglycemia, which may interfere with daily living.

ENDOCRINE EXCESS SYNDROMES

As with deficiency syndromes, excess may occur in primary or secondary forms. A primary disorder occurs when the organ itself produces the excess hormone without stimulation by a trophic gland. An example is primary hyperaldosteronism caused by an autonomous adrenal tumor. An example of a secondary excess syndrome is Cushing's disease, which is caused by increased production of adrenocorticotropic hormone (ACTH) by a pituitary tumor. In this case, there is nothing wrong with the target organ (the adrenal gland)—it is responding as it should to excess trophic hormone. The wide receiver (adrenal gland) is simply obeying the quarterback (pituitary), who has "called the wrong play."

Unlike hormone deficiency (usually caused by autoimmune diseases), hormone excess syndromes are typically caused by tumors (benign or malignant). These tumors typically arise in the organ that normally produces the hormone. Hyperfunctioning tumors may also arise in an organ other than the one normally producing the hormone; these conditions are called paraneoplastic or "out of place" syndromes. We will discuss these syndromes in the final lecture. Autoimmune syndromes only rarely cause endocrine excess. An exception is Graves' disease, where thyroid autoantibodies mimic the trophic hormone (TSH) and result in hyperthyroidism.

Another reason for hormone excess is exogenous administration of the hormone, either intentionally (iatrogenic) or by the patient without the physician's knowledge (factitious). For example, glucocorticoids are commonly used at high doses to treat transplant rejection. Chronic administration results in iatrogenic Cushing's syndrome. An example of factitious hormone use is the person who wishes to lose weight by taking exogenous thyroid hormone, not prescribed by any physician. These cases are often health care workers with psychiatric problems and access to medication.

IMAGING TESTS IN ENDOCRINOLOGY

Plain x-rays (roentgenograms) are inexpensive and simple to perform, but have limited use in endocrinology. At the energy levels used for imaging, x-rays are absorbed to a great extent by molecules containing elements with high atomic numbers (Z, or number of protons in the nucleus). Such molecules appear opaque (white) on x-ray. Iodine (Z = 53) and barium (Z = 56) are relatively heavy elements, which is why they are commonly used as radiocontrast agents. (This use of stable iodine has nothing to do with the uses of its radioactive counterparts.) Molecules containing calcium (Z = 20) also show up well on x-ray (think of bones). Some endocrine disorders are associated with ectopic calcification and may be detected on plain x-ray. Most organic molecules contain large amounts of carbon, oxygen, nitrogen, and hydrogen, with low atomic numbers.

Nuclear medicine imaging studies use radioactive substances that are administered to patients. They may be given orally (e.g., radioiodine), intravenously (technetium sulfur colloid), or inhaled (xenon). The element used is typically a radioactive counterpart (isotope) of a nonradioactive element. For example, ^{123}I and ^{131}I are isotopes of the nonradioactive (stable) ^{127}I. The superscript immediately preceding the chemical symbol indicates the mass number (A), which is the number of protons (Z) plus the number of neutrons. Other elements do not occur in the natural compound but are similar in structure and chemical properties to the natural element. Technetium (^{99m}Tc) is a synthetic element with radioactive properties very suitable for imaging. Its ease of incorporation into numerous compounds and lack of toxicity makes it the "Swiss army knife" of radionuclides. The radioactive element is either administered in its native form or attached to a molecule that mimics the native substance.

Radionuclides may emit radiation in several ways. They may emit nonparticulate energy such as photons (gamma rays), which are essentially high-energy light beams. Gamma radiation occurs after a nuclear event (e.g., beta decay) that leaves the nucleus in an excited state. When the nucleus returns to its unexcited (ground) state, gamma rays are emitted from the nucleus. X-rays are exactly the same as gamma rays except that their origin is the outer electron shells rather than the nucleus when an electron passes from a higher to a lower energy state. Iodine-123 (^{123}I) and technetium are examples of pure gamma emitters.

Some radionuclides emit particulate radiation in addition to gamma rays. The nuclides of clinical interest emit beta (β) particles, which are electrons ejected from the nucleus, resulting in conversion of a neutron to a proton. Beta particles may cause significant tissue destruction, and therefore these elements are less suitable for imaging. They are used when actual destruction of tissue is desired. ^{131}I is a powerful beta emitter used to destroy thyroid tissue in those with hyperthyroidism and thyroid cancer. Heavy nuclides that emit alpha particles (e.g., thorium, uranium) have no clinical use in nuclear medicine.

Radionuclides disintegrate because of the very properties that make them radioactive. The half-life is the amount of time for half of the nuclide to disintegrate. Decay is exponential and the amount present at any time can be calculated if the half-life and original amount of the radionuclide are known:

$$A = A_0 e^{\frac{-0.693t}{t_{1/2}}}$$

where A = activity of the nuclide at the current time; A_0 = original activity of nuclide; t = time elapsed; $t_{1/2}$ = half-life of nuclide; and e = base of the natural logarithm (2.71828...).

The physical amount of a radionuclide is denoted by its activity and is proportional to the number of disintegrations per second. The traditional unit of radionuclide activity is the curie (named after Marie Curie, a prominent nuclear physicist and discoverer of polonium and radium). The amounts used in nuclear medicine are in the range of 1/1000th curie (millicurie, mCi) or 1/1,000,000th curie (microcurie, μCi). Another unit of activity is the becquerel (Bq); 1 mCi = 37 MBq (megabecquerels). The delivered dose of radiation depends on many factors, such as type of energy emitted and energy of the gamma rays, and is beyond the scope of this text. For example, 30 mCi of ^{131}I delivers approximately 100 times as much radiation as 30 mCi of ^{123}I because of the increased energy and particulate emissions of the former.

A radiation counter can detect the amount of gamma radiation emitted. It merely measures the amount of radiation coming from the patient and provides no spatial information. A radionuclide uptake may be calculated using these measurements to provide the fractional amount of nuclide accumulated at a given time. A more complex device, a gamma camera, can produce a two-dimensional image or scan of the organ radiating the energy. Gamma cameras are used to produce thyroid scan images, for example. Although nuclear medicine provides useful functional information, the scan resolution is typically far less than other imaging modalities.

Ultrasound utilizes high-frequency sound waves and takes advantage of their attenuation by various materials. Sound waves are generated by a transducer and placed in contact with the body. The sound is either reflected back to the transducer or absorbed. The distance between the transducer and the reflected echo is calculated by measuring the time between the transmitted wave and the echo. Material that absorbs sound (e.g., air) transmits little or no sound back to the transducer. Very sophisticated images can be obtained by using multiple transducers; high-speed computers collect and interpret the data in a two-dimensional form that can be displayed on a screen.

Unlike nuclear medicine, ultrasound does not expose the patient to ionizing radiation. It also is a "real-time" modality that can be used to guide procedures (e.g., fine-needle aspiration biopsy or insertion of a catheter into a difficult area). The resolution of ultrasound, however, is less than that of MRI (magnetic resonance imaging) or CT (computed tomography). Nor is ultrasound very useful for air-filled cavities (e.g., lung).

Computed tomography (CT) uses conventional x-ray beams to produce high-resolution "cross-sections" of a body part. The patient is placed between the x-ray tube and a series of x-ray detectors, which move in a circular fashion around the patient. After the detectors have completed a full circle around the patient, the data is analyzed by a computer, which reconstructs an image, a virtual "cross-section" of the area of interest. A recent development is the high-resolution (helical or spiral) CT, in which the x-ray tube and detectors move in a helical fashion from one end of the area to the other, resulting in many more data points than conventional CT. Single-photon emission computed tomography (SPECT) is a hybrid of CT and nuclear medicine that uses an administered nuclear source rather than an x-ray beam for the radiation source.

Because of its speed, CT is useful for imaging large body cavities (e.g., chest, abdomen, or pelvis) that contain visceral organs. Iodine-containing contrast agents are often administered. These are contraindicated in those with renal insufficiency. Many patients are allergic and require pretreatment with corticosteroids and antihistamines. These agents also interfere with radioiodine imaging of the thyroid for at least four weeks.

Magnetic resonance imaging (MRI) takes advantage of the effect of hydrogen nuclei when exposed to a strong magnetic field. At rest, the nuclei are oriented at random. When exposed to a magnetic field, the nuclei "polarize" and oscillate at a certain frequency that is unique to each atom. Since the body is about 80% water (H_2O), there is a lot of hydrogen to polarize. Sophisticated computer reconstruction of these faint MR signals results in detailed cross-sectional images of the body. A greater variety of imaging angles is available than with CT. Another advantage is the lack of ionizing radiation. A disadvantage is the relatively long scan times compared to CT. The patient must often be enclosed, which may be difficult for those with claustrophobia. "Open" MRI units now exist in which the patient is only partially enclosed. These devices use weaker magnets, however, and may be less suitable for precise imaging of very small structures such as the pituitary.

Positron emission tomography (PET) uses short-lived radionuclides. A positron is an electron with a positive charge. When a positron and electron strike each other, they are converted to energy by an annihilation reaction, which is detected by sensors. PET has been used primarily to measure cerebral and myocardial blood flow, but shows promise in certain endocrine applications. A disadvantage of PET is the extremely short half-lives of the radionuclides, mandating that they be made at the facility in a cyclotron. Because of the massive expense of a PET system, this imaging modality is limited primarily to large academic medical centers.

EPILOGUE

This lecture has laid the framework for discussion of the endocrine system. Hopefully, you now have a basic idea of how the different systems fit together. In the next several lectures, we will examine each of the "players" in detail. Finally, we will discuss disorders of multiple endocrine glands in the last lecture.

PITUITARY AND HYPOTHALAMUS

REVIEW

Let's quickly review the first lecture. We learned that complex multicellular organisms require a way to regulate bodily functions by communicating between cells. This is accomplished by means of the endocrine system, in which a substance (hormone) secreted by one type of cell may have an effect on a cell far away, in a different part of the body. Hormones are necessary for cellular communication and regulation. If hormone levels get "out of whack," the body does not function at optimal efficiency. Most hormones are proteins made of tens to hundreds of amino acids. Others are modified amino acids (catecholamines, iodothyronines) or derivatives of cholesterol (steroids). Glycoproteins are a special type of protein hormone to which large sugar molecules are attached.

Each hormone has a desired effect on a target cell. The effect may be stimulatory (to cause the cell to produce a substance, usually a protein), or inhibitory (to inhibit production of the substance). Production of this substance in the target cell takes place in the nucleus. Some hormones go to the nucleus directly and have their effect there. Other hormones attach to the cell membrane and trigger production of one or more second messengers that travel to the nucleus and produce the desired effect. A multiple messenger "cascade" allows extremely low amounts of these hormones to have a significant effect. Some hormones travel in serum bound to carrier proteins—others travel in the free state.

Understanding hormonal regulation is key to understanding endocrinology. Most hormones have another hormone that regulates their secretion. Those that stimulate a hormone's secretion are called trophic hormones. Those that inhibit are called inhibitory hormones. A trophic hormone has a target gland and once the target gland hormone reaches a normal level, feedback inhibition on the trophic gland keeps levels from becoming too high. In a way, the target hormone becomes a sort of indirect inhibitory hormone. All endocrine disorders result from disruption of the normal feedback mechanisms.

Endocrine hypofunction is common and typically is caused by an abnormal or absent gland (a primary deficiency). Autoimmune gland destruction is the most common cause of primary endocrine hypofunction. Less common are the secondary and tertiary causes of hypofunction, in which deficient trophic hormones result in inadequate target gland function. A target organ's resistance to the trophic hormone may also cause hypofunction. In most cases of organ hypofunction, we try to replace the native hormone. However, this is not possible or practical in some instances.

In contrast to organ hypofunction, most cases of endocrine hyperfunction are caused by tumors, while autoimmune causes of hyperfunction are rare. Another cause of endocrine excess is the exogenous administration of a hormone (e.g., thyroid hormone or glucocorticoids).

Some hormones may be measured in their basal state. Many, however, are secreted periodically, and random measurement may not be useful. When endocrine hypofunction is suspected, we often perform a stimulatory test by giving the trophic hormone to the patient. The response to the stimulus is then measured. If we suspect endocrine excess, an inhibitory test is performed by administering an inhibitor of the hormone.

Many imaging tests are useful in endocrinology. Plain x-rays are inexpensive but have limited value in endocrinology. Nuclear medicine involves the administration of radioactive substances that are assimilated into compounds inside the body. The radiation source therefore is the patient, and radiation counts and/or images may be obtained to assess function. Most nuclear medicine studies in endocrinology use radioactive iodine. One type of radioiodine is very useful for imaging. Another type is more useful for destroying thyroid tissue. Technetium, a synthetic element, is also useful in nuclear medicine.

CT (computed tomography) utilizes conventional x-rays to produce cross-sections of an organ. MRI (magnetic resonance imaging) uses powerful magnetic fields to produce cross-sectional images as well. MRI provides better resolution of some endocrine structures (e.g., pituitary) than does CT. Ultrasound utilizes the attenuation of high-frequency sound waves by an organ to provide a real-time image. Advantages of MRI and ultrasound include the absence of ionizing radiation.

PITUITARY AND HYPOTHALAMUS

In this chapter we will discuss the "master glands": the pituitary and hypothalamus. In our football team analogy, they are sort of like the "quarterback" that directs the rest of the glands. (Not every gland is controlled by the pituitary and hypothalamus; think of these other glands as "special team" glands.) In fact, the pituitary and hypothalamus tend to function together as one unit, which we will call the hypothalamic-pituitary axis or HPA, and which serves to integrate the central nervous system and the endocrine system. Most of the "classical" endocrine glands are under control of the HPA.

The pituitary is a small gland that lies in a part of the skull called the sella turcica, at the base of the skull. It is divided into the anterior lobe (adenohypophysis) and the posterior lobe (neurohypophysis). The anterior lobe cells manufacture what we normally think of as the pituitary hormones. Their secretion is influenced by hypothalamic hormones that travel to the anterior lobe via a humoral system called the hypophyseal portal system.

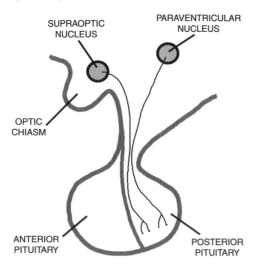

The anterior pituitary makes hormones that control specific glands, which include:

ACTH (adrenocorticotrophic hormone or corticotropin)—adrenal cortex
GH (growth hormone or somatotropin)—bone and muscle
PRL (prolactin)—milk-producing glands of breast
TSH (thyroid-stimulating hormone or thyrotropin)—thyroid
LH (luteinizing hormone) and FSH (follicle-stimulating hormone)—ovaries and testes

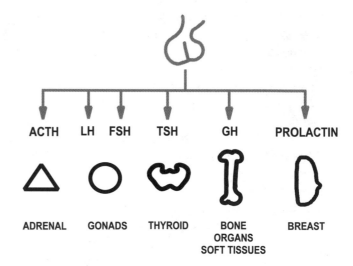

The hypothalamus is a group of neurons in the midbrain that secretes a variety of substances. The hormones can be divided into two types. The first are those that stimulate the anterior pituitary gland to produce its hormones. The hypothalamus makes a hormone that stimulates production of each of the hormones above (except for prolactin, which has no well-defined stimulatory hormone). The hypothalamus also makes inhibitory hormones for some of the anterior pituitary hormones above. The hypothalamic hormones and their actions include:

TRH (thyrotropin releasing hormone)—stimulates TSH secretion
GHRH (growth hormone–releasing hormone)—stimulates GH secretion
GnRH (gonadotropin-releasing hormone)—stimulates FSH and LH secretion
CRH (corticotropin-releasing hormone)—stimulates ACTH secretion

PRH (prolactin-releasing hormone)—stimulates prolactin secretion
Dopamine—inhibits prolactin secretion
Somatostatin—inhibits GH and TSH secretion

Traditionally, it has been felt that prolactin had no well-defined stimulatory hormone, only an inhibitory one (dopamine). Recently, however, scientists have discovered a hypothalamic peptide that appears to increase prolactin secretion by the pituitary, hence the name PRH or prolactin-releasing hormone.

The posterior lobe can be envisioned simply as an extension of the hypothalamus, and the second type of hypothalamic hormones are those that are secreted by the posterior pituitary gland. These include antidiuretic hormone (ADH), important in the body's conservation of water. The other, oxytocin, helps uterine muscle contract during childbirth. It is of no clinical significance in males.

GROWTH HORMONE

When many people think of the pituitary, they think of growth hormone and its disorders, such as pituitary gigantism and dwarfism. Growth hormone is not essential to life in the adult, but is necessary for normal growth and development. It has a direct effect on certain tissues, such as increasing protein synthesis fatty acid release. It is in fact a "stress" hormone and increased during times of stress. Its most striking effects, however, are those on bone and cartilage, where it promotes linear growth. This is not a direct effect of GH, but is mediated through a substance called insulin-like growth factor I (IGF-I). An older name for this molecule is somatomedin C. It is called insulin-like growth factor because it has some effects similar to insulin. GH stimulates the liver to produce IGF-I, which then stimulates bone and cartilage to grow.

Like many pituitary hormones, GH is secreted in cyclical fashion with peak levels occurring during sleep. Many factors increase or decrease secretion. Growth hormone is a stress hormone, so things such as exercise increase its concentration. Growth hormone tends to promote glucose release, and low blood glucose (hypoglycemia) also is a stimulus for its secretion. In contrast, high blood glucose (hyperglycemia) inhibits its release.

Now is a good time to talk about normal growth and development. For most people, growth is normal and there are no concerns. For others, however, growth is abnormal and we need to distinguish abnormal from normal growth and development. One way is by constructing a growth curve. This is a simple graph made by plotting height versus age. These are usually plotted on graph paper with normal standards for boys and girls. The middle line represents the 50th percentile; the upper and lower lines, 95th and 5th percentiles, respectively.

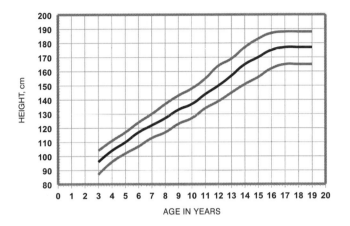

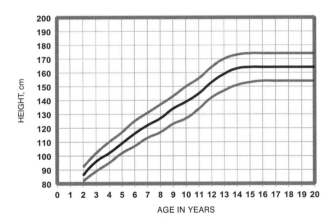

Although these curves give us some useful information, more information is found by constructing a growth velocity curve. This is a little bit more complex than a simple growth curve. In the growth velocity curve, we first must determine the rate of growth at each growth point, plotting against age. For example, if a child grew from 140 to 144 cm in 6 months the rate of growth would be 4 cm per 6 months or 8 cm/year. The growth rate is highest during infancy, falls off steadily, and then increases again at puberty (the "growth spurt"). As final adult height is attained, the growth velocity falls to zero.

A common question is how to estimate how tall a child will be. This is not always possible to estimate exactly, since many factors play into final height. Because height is normally distributed, any set of given

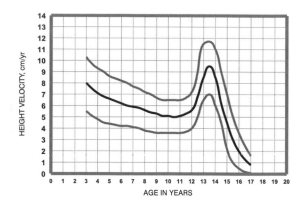

parents may have children that are either taller or shorter than they are.

SHORT STATURE AND GROWTH HORMONE DEFICIENCY

The most typical growth-related complaint is short stature. Our society tends to place emphasis on height and it is natural that everyone wants to be tall. Height, like weight, intelligence, and many other parameters, is normally distributed; it stands to reason that a small percentage of patients will fall at the lower end, just as a few will fall at the higher end. It is important to distinguish normal from pathological short stature. The most common cause of short stature is constitutional short stature, which is just a variation from normal for the population. It stands to reason that short parents tend to produce short children. When we look at the growth curves for patients with constitutional short stature, they normally stay at the same percentile throughout their entire growth. For example, a boy who is at the 5th percentile when he is four years old will probably be at the 5th percentile when he is 12 years old, unless there is a pathological problem. Children that cross percentiles raise a red flag for a pathological condition.

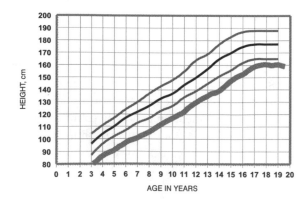

What are some pathological causes of short stature? Patients with growth hormone deficiency certainly will have short stature. This is a type of short stature that is proportional, that is, he or she looks normal except for being small. Mothers that use drugs or have intrauterine infections (such as rubella) may have children with short stature. An interesting form of short stature occurs in children who are deprived of attention and affection. This is called psychosocial dwarfism and may be reversible if the child is removed from the dysfunctional environment. Children with severe, chronic medical conditions (e.g., renal failure) may develop short stature. Drugs that inhibit growth (e.g., glucocorticoids) may cause short stature if given in childhood.

Some types of short stature are not proportional. The most common example is achondroplastic dwarfism. In this condition, the face, hands, feet, face, and trunk are normal in size, but the limbs are disproportionately short. There is no treatment for this disorder.

Growth hormone deficiency is treated with injections of GH. It must usually be given daily, although a depot GH preparation is now available. Years ago, GH was scarce, as it had to be procured from cadaver pituitary glands. Fortunately, growth hormone can now be manufactured using genetic engineering technology, ensuring a limitless supply of growth hormone. However, it still is very expensive to produce and treatment may cost $30,000 per year or more.

TALL STATURE AND GH EXCESS

Tall stature is generally not a cause for concern because society traditionally views it as desirable. As with short stature, the most common cause of tall stature is constitutional tall stature occurring in the children of tall parents.

Pathologic causes of tall stature are rare. Gigantism occurs when excess growth hormone is present during childhood or puberty. This results in accelerated bone growth and excessive tall stature. These patients eventually develop disfigurement because of the effects of growth hormone on the face, hands, and feet. The tallest giant on record, Robert Wadlow, was 8 feet 11 inches tall (272 cm) and weighed 490 pounds (220 kg) at the time of his death at age 22. Excess growth hormone has many adverse effects on the body, and most giants have a decreased life expectancy.

If you watch a professional basketball game, you might wonder how many of these men and women have gigantism, since the average height of a male pro basketball player is approximately 6 feet 8 inches (203 cm). Many women players exceed 6 feet 4 inches (193 cm). You might be surprised to learn that these men and women simply have constitutional tall stature. If you were to measure the growth hormone levels of a professional basketball player and compare those to persons with constitutional short stature, you would find similar levels. There simply are genetic differences in the expression of height that are independent of growth hormone levels. Giants typically are very poor athletes. Despite their large bulk and muscle mass, their muscles are actually weaker than normal and they are prone to develop problems with arthritis and cardiac disease.

For a patient to develop gigantism, the growth hormone excess obviously has to occur before the patient has finished growing. A more common disease occurs when growth hormone excess is present in adulthood. This is called acromegaly and is so named because of the enlargement of the face, hands, and feet in these patients. Since these patients are adults when the growth hormone excess starts, the long bones cannot grow further, so their height remains the same. They do, however, become disfigured, because of the other effects on the hands, face, and feet. Acromegaly also may result in enlargement of organs such as the heart, which can lead to cardiac disease and even death. In addition, growth hormone in large concentrations may cause diabetes. This might seem counterintuitive, since we discussed that growth hormone causes the production of insulin-like growth factor (IGF-I) by the liver. Although IGF-I does have some insulin-like actions, the anti-insulin effects of excess growth hormone far outweigh this effect of IGF-I, and glucose intolerance results. High blood pressure (hypertension) also may result. Acromegalics often develop arthritis and visual field defects due to compression of the optic nerve by the large pituitary tumor.

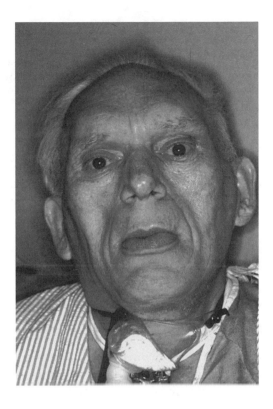

As we have discussed, random measurement of pituitary hormones is often not very useful. When we suspect endocrine excess, we typically do a suppressive study. A natural inhibitor of growth hormone secretion is hyperglycemia, so we commonly perform what is called a glucose tolerance test to evaluate growth hormone excess. Growth hormone is measured before and after the ingestion of a glucose-containing drink (100 grams). In normal patients, GH suppresses below a certain level (<2 ng/mL). Patients with either acromegaly or gigantism do not suppress, thus confirming the diagnosis. IGF-I levels are also elevated in acromegaly and/or gigantism.

Growth hormone-secreting tumors can be treated in several ways. One way is to perform surgery and remove the tumor. Smaller tumors can be removed by a transsphenoidal approach (through the roof of the mouth). Larger tumors must be removed via a transfrontal approach (through the forehead).

A natural inhibitor of growth hormone secretion is the hypothalamic hormone somatostatin. A synthetic hormone, octreotide, is a long-acting analog of somatostatin and in fact inhibits growth hormone-secreting tumors. This medication is given by injection and works so well that sometimes surgery is not necessary. In severe cases not responsive to either surgery or octreotide, radiation therapy is used to destroy the tumor.

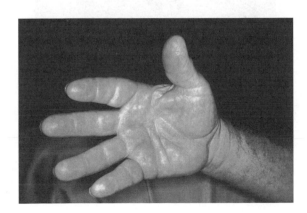

PROLACTIN

We will next discuss prolactin because it is related somewhat to growth hormone—both are derived from a similar precursor and produced by the same cell type. The similarity ends there, however, as they have vastly different physiological functions. The function of prolactin is to stimulate proliferation of lactation (mammary) glands, which results in milk production after birth of an infant. During pregnancy, the increased estrogen levels result in increased prolactin secretion and ductal proliferation in the breast. In the postpartum period, lactation results. Another consequence of hyperprolactinemia is decreased gonadotropin secretion. Prolactin levels are typically very high after parturition, and this in fact prevents another pregnancy from occurring until the infant has been weaned from breast milk. This might not be very important today, but it was very important in more primitive times when reliable methods of birth control were not available. It is detrimental for females of any species to be continuously pregnant, so prolactin plays a secondary role in mammals by preventing the family from becoming excessively large. Men do not really need prolactin, and no clinical syndrome results from its deficiency.

Thus far we have limited our discussion to physiologic prolactin secretion. What happens when prolactin is pathologically secreted? Let us recall what prolactin does. When prolactin is secreted in excess, it suppresses the gonadotropins (LH and FSH), which then results in decreased gonadal function. As mentioned above, this results in amenorrhea (lack of menses) in the female. Prolactin excess in the male results in hypogonadism and infertility. Unlike the female, however, there is no normal physiologic mechanism that results in hyperprolactinemia in the male. Women with excess prolactin may lactate. When this occurs in the absence of pregnancy it is called galactorrhea (galactose is the sugar found in milk). Men only rarely have galactorrhea because of the high estrogen levels needed for milk production. The most common cause of pathologic prolactin secretion is a prolactin secreting pituitary tumor, which are called prolactinomas.

Fortunately, we have an easy way to treat these pituitary tumors. Since dopamine is a normal antagonist of prolactin, we may administer a synthetic analog of dopamine that inhibits prolactin secretion. The most commonly used drug is bromocriptine, which reduces prolactin levels to normal in many cases. Once prolactin levels have normalized, the adverse clinical effects of hyperprolactinemia disappear. Very large tumors not responsive to medical therapy may be treated with either surgery or radiation therapy. Fortunately, these treatments are necessary only in a minority of cases.

Many medications can cause hyperprolactinemia. These include many commonly used antidepressants and other drugs for psychiatric disorders. Another common condition that can result in hyperprolactinemia is primary hypothyroidism. In this disorder, the thyroid itself is damaged and cannot respond to normal TSH stimulation. TSH is then produced in large amounts in response to increased TRH (thyrotropin-releasing hormone) secretion from the hypothalamus. TRH appears to increase prolactin as well as TSH secretion. This may occur to such a degree that significant hyperprolactinemia and its consequences (galactorrhea and hypogonadism) may result. Hypothyroidism should therefore be excluded in all patients with hyperprolactinemia. Prolactin levels return to normal after treatment of the hypothyroidism.

PITUITARY TUMORS

Let us now shift our focus to pituitary tumors in general. Pituitary tumors may be classified as microadenomas (<1 cm in diameter) or macroadenomas (>1 cm in diameter).

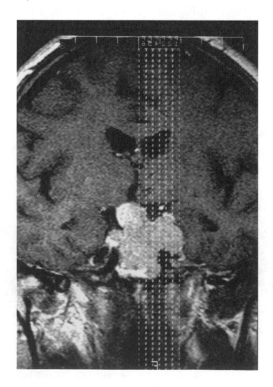

Some pituitary tumors produce hormones, such as growth hormone or prolactin. Other tumors are non-functional (i.e., they do not make any hormones). These nonfunctional or nonsecretory pituitary tumors account for approximately 10% of all pituitary tumors. They may be found on a CT (computed tomogram) or an MRI (magnetic resonance imaging) scan done for another reason. Although these tumors do not produce any hormones, they may cause damage because of their size. Pituitary tumors may cause headache and/or visual field defects and potentially hypopituitarism. The pituitary lies right above the optic chiasm (where the optic nerves cross on the way to the eyes). Because nonfunctional tumors are non-hormone-secreting, they do not respond to specific medical treatment like those that are hormone-secreting. Large tumors may need to be reduced surgically or with radiotherapy.

HYPOPITUITARISM

Hypopituitarism is a condition resulting from the deficiency of one or more pituitary hormones; panhypopituitarism is the deficiency of all pituitary hormones. The most common cause is destruction of the gland by a pituitary tumor. Surgery and irradiation of the pituitary also commonly cause hypopituitarism. Severe head trauma can damage the pituitary stalk. Tumors that destroy the hypothalamus result in hypothalamic hormone deficiency and hypopituitarism. This is called "tertiary" hormone deficiency.

What are the clinical consequences of panhypopituitarism? Some of these hormones are necessary for life. The body cannot survive without thyroid hormone and adrenocortical hormones, so without TSH and ACTH death occurs. Fortunately, thyroid hormone (thyroxine) and cortisol (hydrocortisone) are inexpensive and easily absorbed orally. Gonadotropin (LH and FSH) deficiency, although not life-threatening, results in hypogonadism and infertility. Deficiency of growth hormone in childhood results in an adult with proportional short stature. Growth hormone deficiency in adults has no devastating consequences, although recent research suggests that growth hormone plays a role in maintaining normal bone and muscle metabolism. Adults who lack growth hormone tend to become less muscular and have a greater proportion of fat. Some adults with GH deficiency are now treated. Prolactin deficiency has no clinical consequences except

for the lack of postpartum lactation. This hardly is life threatening in industrialized countries, as commercial infant formulas are readily available. One interesting cause of panhypopituitarism occurs in the postpartum period in women who experience severe postpartum hemorrhage. This condition, called Sheehan's syndrome, results in pituitary damage and hypopituitarism, including the inability to lactate. Hormone replacement is necessary in these women.

Pituitary (secondary) hypothyroidism is treated by administration of synthetic thyroid hormone (thyroxine). This is the same treatment as for primary hypothyroidism. However, we monitor the treatment differently. As we will learn in the thyroid lecture, we monitor primary hypothyroidism treatment by measuring the serum TSH, and the goal is to keep it in the normal range. TSH, however is not a reliable indicator of thyroid hormone status in secondary (or tertiary) hypothyroidism, since TSH is already deficient. Instead of monitoring TSH, we must measure peripheral hormone (T4 or T3) levels.

Treatment of hypogonadism involves replacement of sex steroids. In women, estrogen is easily replaced orally, which is the preferred method of administration. Estrogen may also be administered as a transdermal patch. Testosterone is metabolized rapidly by the liver and is therefore not acceptable as an oral medication. Testosterone must be administered by intramuscular injection or by transdermal patch or gel.

One interesting difference between primary and secondary (pituitary) hypogonadism is that, in theory, fertility may be restored in the latter. Fertility is impossible in primary hypogonadism since the gonad is permanently damaged. With secondary hypogonadism, however, the gonad is structurally intact but does not work properly because of inadequate stimulation. We can, therefore, administer the gonadotropins themselves, which stimulate the gonads to work properly. This is much easier to accomplish in men than women, because of the complexity of the female reproductive cycle.

Pituitary apoplexy is a serious endocrine emergency. This is caused by spontaneous hemorrhage into the pituitary, which results in pituitary damage and hypopituitarism. These patients usually present with severe headache, blurred vision, and confusion. This constitutes an emergency and requires prompt treatment with glucocorticoids and thyroid hormone (since these hormones are necessary for life).

POSTERIOR PITUITARY

ANTIDIURETIC HORMONE

The posterior pituitary hormones, antidiuretic hormone, and oxytocin are produced in the supraoptic and paraventricular nuclei of the hypothalamus and travel to the posterior pituitary by means of nerve fibers. Antidiuretic hormone (ADH, arginine vasopressin) is of great importance in humans; its major function is to help the body regulate water metabolism. Increased ADH levels increase water reabsorption by the kidney; decreased ADH levels cause increased water loss through the kidneys. This mechanism can be advantageous in several circumstances. Imagine a person who is running a marathon. This person may become very dehydrated, and ADH levels increase in an effort to hold on to whatever water is present in the body. In contrast, visualize a person who drank too much water. ADH levels decrease so that the body can excrete this excess water. If this does not happen, he or she may become water intoxicated, which can lead to problems such as low sodium levels (hyponatremia) and confusion.

DIABETES INSIPIDUS

Diabetes insipidus (DI) is a disorder in which antidiuretic hormone is either deficient or does not have appropriate action. (It is not related to diabetes mellitus, which is a disorder of glucose metabolism.) These patients cannot hold on to appropriate amounts of water and therefore urinate quite frequently, sometimes passing over 10 liters of urine per day. They must constantly drink water to replace the amount that is lost in the urine, and this can lead to significant lifestyle disruptions. Patients with diabetes insipidus typically keep water at the bedside so they have something to drink when they wake up. They are unable to take any long trips without having to stop at the bathroom quite often. They also have all the restroom locations at the local shopping malls memorized. If your patient with diabetes insipidus must wait very long in your office, you'll probably see him or her make several trips to the drinking fountain and the bathroom.

There are two types of DI. The first results from a deficiency of ADH, and is called central or neurogenic DI. This often results from some type of pituitary or hypothalamic damage secondary to trauma or surgery.

It also may present for no apparent reason (idiopathic). The second type of diabetes insipidus is called nephrogenic DI and is a hormone resistance syndrome rather than a deficiency syndrome. This means that adequate amounts of ADH are produced, but the kidney is unresponsive to it. This condition results from a variety of renal disorders, and is frequently seen in patients on lithium therapy for psychiatric disorders.

Patients with diabetes insipidus can survive as long as they have free access to water and have an intact thirst mechanism. If the patient is denied free access to water (e.g., if they are hospitalized for an acute illness) they may become dehydrated. This type of lifestyle however is very disruptive, and therapy is recommended to most patients with diabetes insipidus. Central diabetes insipidus is easily treated with the synthetic ADH derivative desmopressin. ADH itself is typically not used because it is degraded very rapidly and has other undesirable effects such as increasing blood pressure (hence the name vasopressin). Desmopressin is very long lasting and is devoid of these other effects. Desmopressin may be given as a nasal spray or as oral tablets. Patients without an intact thirst mechanism may develop problems if they drink too little water (they become dehydrated) or if they drink too much water (becoming water intoxicated).

There are several medications that augment the action of ADH. These medications are useful in patients who make a little bit of ADH but are ineffective in those who don't make ADH at all. These medications include chlorpropamide (an oral agent also used for type 2 diabetes), carbamazepine (an anticonvulsant), and clofibrate (a lipid-lowering medication).

Nephrogenic diabetes insipidus is less easily treated. Since the patient already makes adequate amounts of ADH, giving extra ADH does not help since they are resistant to it. Some diuretics enhance free water absorption (e.g., hydrochlorothiazide and amiloride) and are useful in many patients.

There are conditions other than DI that can result in polyuria and polydipsia. The most significant to exclude is diabetes mellitus. Another relatively common cause is psychogenic polydipsia (compulsive water drinking). This is a condition in which the patient consumes too much water (often >10 gallons per day). Many of these patients have underlying psychiatric problems and often take medications that cause dry mouth, thus prompting them to drink too much water. Psychogenic polydipsia is treated by restricting water intake.

SIADH

Bad things can also happen when the body has too much ADH; excess ADH results in a disorder exactly the opposite of diabetes insipidus, called the syndrome of inappropriate antidiuretic hormone (SIADH). These patients present with hyponatremia (low sodium levels), are by definition euvolemic (i.e., not fluid overloaded from renal or cardiac failure), and have no other endocrine abnormality (hypothyroidism and adrenal insufficiency can cause hyponatremia). Hyponatremia in SIADH may cause confusion, coma, seizures, and even death in severe cases.

A common cause of SIADH is malignancy. Certain tumors such as small-cell lung carcinoma commonly make neuroendocrine peptides such as ADH. Patients with head trauma may experience release of ADH from the hypothalamus. SIADH may also be caused by non-malignant lung conditions (e.g., pneumonia). Several medications can cause SIADH. Patients taking chlorpropamide, carbamazepine, or clofibrate (all of which potentiate ADH action and thus can be used in the treatment of partial central diabetes insipidus) may develop SIADH. Opioid analgesics such as morphine may potentiate ADH action and result in hyponatremia. At times, no cause for the SIADH can be found (idiopathic). SIADH may be distinguished from primary polydipsia (water intoxication) since ADH levels are inappropriately high in the former, and suppressed in the latter.

The first way to treat SIADH is to treat any underlying condition such as malignancy. The next step is generally to restrict the patient's fluids. If this is unsuccessful, a medication called demeclocycline may be used. This negates the effect of ADH on the kidney and restores normal function.

OXYTOCIN

Oxytocin stimulates milk ejection from mammary glands and therefore plays a vital role in lactation. It also stimulates uterine contraction and aids in delivery of the fetus at parturition. Labor can occur in the absence of oxytocin, but it proceeds more slowly. Oxytocin is often given during labor to help with uterine contractions and to decrease postpartum bleeding. Deficiency of oxytocin has no clinical consequences in women who are not giving birth or lactating.

THE THYROID

REVIEW

Let us now review what we learned in the last lecture. We learned about the "quarterback" of our team—the pituitary and hypothalamus, which essentially function together as one unit called the hypothalamic-pituitary axis (HPA).

The pituitary is a small gland that is divided into the anterior and posterior lobes. The anterior pituitary makes hormones such as ACTH, growth hormone, prolactin, TSH, and the gonadotropins (LH and FSH), which control specific glands. The posterior pituitary is actually an extension of the brain. Hormones secreted by this organ include antidiuretic hormone (ADH, vasopressin) and oxytocin.

Growth hormone (GH) is not essential for life in the adult, but is necessary for normal growth in children and adolescents. It has a direct effect on some tissues, but its main effects are mediated by a molecule called insulin-like growth factor I (IGF-I), which is made in the liver. Deficiency of growth hormone results in short stature in children, and may be treated with synthetic growth hormone. Growth hormone therapy has also been shown to provide benefits for adults with GH deficiency. Short stature is a common presenting complaint to an endocrinologist. Most children with short stature have constitutional short stature (e.g., a child of short parents).

Like short stature, most cases of tall stature have no pathologic cause—the most common cause is constitutional tall stature. Growth hormone excess in childhood results in gigantism. Many patients with gigantism are seven feet tall or more (although most people seven feet tall are not giants). Growth hormone excess in adults results in a condition called acromegaly, which causes disfigurement with increased growth of the facial bones, hands, and feet. Growth hormone excess is usually caused by a pituitary tumor.

The hormone prolactin is necessary for normal lactation in females, and plays no significant role in males. Increased prolactin (hyperprolactinemia) may result from a variety of causes. A common cause is a pituitary tumor, although medications may cause hyperprolactinemia. Galactorrhea is the presence of milk in the absence of pregnancy and is a common presenting complaint of hyperprolactinemia in women. Hypogonadism may occur in both men and women with hyperprolactinemia.

Pituitary tumors may produce hormones or may be nonfunctional. Tumors that are very large may cause endocrine effects by destroying the pituitary itself, causing hypopituitarism. Panhypopituitarism is the deficiency of all pituitary hormones. Other causes of hypopituitarism include pituitary surgery and irradiation. Hypothalamic destruction results in hypopituitarism. Panhypopituitarism may result in death due to deficiency of ACTH and TSH, but this may be treated by the administration of synthetic corticosteroids and thyroid hormone. Deficiencies of the other hormones do not result in death but may result in significant morbidity.

Antidiuretic hormone (ADH, arginine vasopressin) is the major hormone of the posterior pituitary. It is important in regulating the body's fluid balance. ADH increases water retention by the kidney. Decreased levels therefore result in increased water loss. Central or neurogenic diabetes insipidus (DI) is a condition in which the pituitary makes too little antidiuretic hormone. These patients cannot hold on to water and have incessant thirst and urination. This condition is easily treated by administration of antidiuretic hormone. Another cause of diabetes insipidus occurs when the body is resistant to antidiuretic hormone. This condition is less easily treated. Persons with DI must be distinguished from those with psychogenic polydipsia (water intoxication), who simply drink too much water.

The opposite of diabetes insipidus is SIADH (syndrome of inappropriate antidiuretic hormone). This syndrome is most commonly caused by tumors that make ADH, but may also be caused by other conditions or medications. These patients have too much water and may develop severe electrolyte disturbances. Restricting water intake and administering drugs that inhibit the action of antidiuretic hormone can treat this condition.

THE THYROID

The largest endocrine organ is the thyroid. It has two lobes, an isthmus (middle), and a small embryonic remnant, the pyramidal lobe. The normal thyroid weighs about 20 grams, but may become enlarged to many times this size in disease states.

The thyroid is important for many reasons. Thyroid hormones are necessary for life, and have a variety of functions. They increase the body's metabolism, resulting in increased oxygen consumption, heart contractility, intestinal motility, bone remodeling, and degradation of many substances (e.g., cholesterol, medications, other hormones). In our analogy of the endocrine system as a football team, the thyroid is like the linemen who help the other players catch passes and move downfield. Without enough thyroid hormone, the body basically "slows down" and becomes sluggish (kind of like playing a videotape in slow motion). Too much thyroid hormone results in a stimulated individual (like playing a videotape too fast).

THYROID HORMONES

The major molecule made by the thyroid is the hormone 3,5,3',5'-tetraiodothyronine or thyroxine (T4). T4 is made from two modified tyrosine molecules hooked together with four iodine atoms attached (hence the name T4). T4 is highly protein bound, and for a hormone has a very long serum half-life (one week). In the blood, T4 loses one iodine atom, and the hormone triiodothyronine or T3 is formed. This new hormone is much more potent than T4. You might ask, then, why doesn't the thyroid just make T3 instead of T4? The reason is that T4 lasts much longer in the blood than T3

(seven days versus one day). T4 therefore serves as a storage reservoir for later conversion to T3.

3,5,3',5-L-tetraiodothyronine (thyroxine, T4)

3,5,3'-L-triiodothyronine (T3)

The stimulus for thyroid hormone secretion is TSH (thyroid-stimulating hormone), produced by the pituitary gland. (TSH is not properly called a thyroid hormone because it is made in the pituitary gland.)

The functional unit of the thyroid where thyroid hormones are synthesized is the follicle, which is under strict control by TSH. Thyroid hormone synthesis starts when iodine atoms are brought into the follicular cell by means of a process called trapping. Since the iodine content inside the follicle must be much greater than outside the follicle, this requires active transport (i.e., against a concentration gradient). Once the iodine atoms are inside the thyroid follicle, they are activated to an oxidized state by thyroid peroxidase. While this is going on, the protein thyroglobulin is being synthesized in the thyroid follicle and tyrosine residues are attached to this. After this backbone is assembled, the activated iodine molecules are incorporated into the thyroglobulin molecule by a process called organification. After some rearrangement, the result is T4 attached to the thyroglobulin molecule. The resulting T4-thyroglobulin complex is then moved to the proteinaceous substance in the center of the follicle called the colloid where it may be stored for long periods of time. The thyroid is somewhat unique in that it can store its hormone for weeks at a time unlike most other glands, which synthesize their hormone as needed.

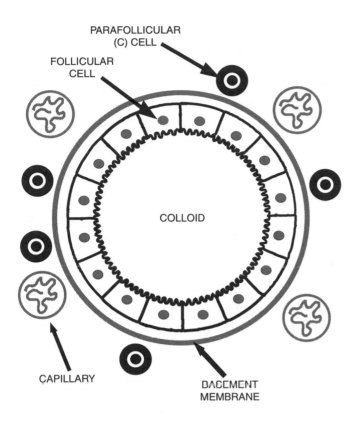

PARAFOLLICULAR (C) CELL

FOLLICULAR CELL

COLLOID

CAPILLARY

BASEMENT MEMBRANE

When thyroid hormone is needed, the T4-thyroglobulin complex passes from the colloid into the follicular cell and T4 is cleaved from the complex, yielding T4 molecules that flow into the bloodstream. In the peripheral circulation T4 is then deiodinated to T3, the active hormone.

EFFECTS OF THYROID HORMONE

Unlike many hormones that have effects only on certain organs, the thyroid hormones have effects in almost all tissues of the body. A primary role of thyroid hormone is to increase energy expenditure and thermogenesis. Hence, persons with thyroid hormone deficiency complain of cold intolerance.

Protein, carbohydrate, and lipid metabolism are affected by the iodothyronines. Low doses of thyroid hormones promote glycogen synthesis, whereas larger doses stimulate glycogen breakdown. Intestinal absorption of glucose is also accelerated by thyroid hormone. Cholesterol metabolism is depressed in thyroid hormone deficiency, and levels rise in those with hypothyroidism, leading to increased risk of atherosclerosis.

THYROID REGULATION

How is homeostasis maintained? Our quarterback the pituitary gland plays a major role in regulation of the thyroid gland. When T4 and T3 levels become too low, the pituitary and hypothalamus detect this, and increased TRH and TSH production results. Increased TSH then results in the return of normal T4 levels by increasing synthesis through any mechanisms outlined above. The opposite occurs when T4 levels get too high. TRH and TSH levels diminish, with resultant decreased hormone synthesis and return of levels to normal.

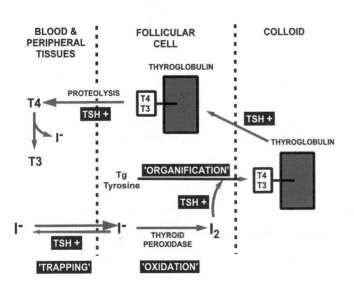

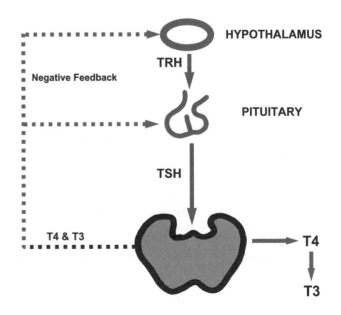

As we learned from the overview chapter, only the free or unbound portion (about 0.04% of the total hormone for T4) is biologically active (the bound portion is not). The conventional T4 or T3 assay measures the total hormone level. In most cases this is not clinically significant. There are some conditions that change the concentration of binding proteins without changing the total level. Measuring the free or unbound portion eliminates these problems and is often preferred to measuring the total levels.

There are other commonly used tests of thyroid function in addition to the serum hormone assays. A thyroid scan is performed by giving a known amount of radioactive iodine to the patient in oral form. The patient returns the next day, and a scan image of the thyroid is produced with a large device called a gamma camera. Although the term gamma camera sounds ominous, this device is only a large camera that takes pictures of gamma rays, just as your film camera takes pictures of visible light. This procedure yields a low-resolution, two-dimensional picture of the thyroid that can point out structural abnormalities such as thyroid nodules. Another piece of information obtained from this study is the thyroid uptake, which is the fractional amount of radioiodine that has accumulated in the patient's thyroid at 24 hours (accounting, of course for the amount that is lost by natural decay). A normal uptake is about 20%–35% in the United States. This amount varies depending on iodine intake in the diet.

Radioiodine uptake often correlates with thyroid hormone output. Those with very low uptake values may have hypothyroidism, while those with high values may have hyperthyroidism. This is not always the case, however! Serum biochemistry rather than radioiodine uptake should be used to establish thyroid hormone status.

There are two types of radioactive iodine used in nuclear medicine, iodine 123 (^{123}I) and iodine 131 (^{131}I). All isotopes of iodine have the same number of protons ($Z = 53$ for iodine) and hence the same chemical properties, but different neutron (N) and mass (A) numbers. ^{123}I has a very short half-life, emits low energy radiation, and is primarily used for thyroid scans. ^{131}I emits high-energy gamma rays plus β particles (electrons) and is not routinely used for scanning, but rather when actual destruction of the thyroid is desired (e.g., in thyroid cancer and hyperthyroidism).

The thyroid ultrasound is another commonly performed procedure. This is noninvasive and exposes the patient to no radiation. Ultrasound gives detailed cross-sections of the thyroid, revealing anatomic structures that cannot be seen with radioiodine scans. No imaging procedure can accurately distinguish benign from malignant lesions, however.

HYPOTHYROIDISM

We will discuss hypothyroidism first in our thyroid lecture because it is by far the most common thyroid disease and probably the most common endocrine disease. Hypothyroidism is a condition in which the thyroid hormone levels are too low. Most often, hypothyroidism is primary in nature (i.e., due to failure of the thyroid gland itself). Less commonly, hypothyroidism may be secondary (due to pituitary failure) or tertiary (due to hypothalamic dysfunction).

The most common cause of primary hypothyroidism in the United States is a disease called Hashimoto's thyroiditis. Like many endocrine deficiency disorders, it is an autoimmune disease (caused by antithyroid antibodies) that results in inefficient hormonogenesis and gland destruction. It is one of the most common autoimmune diseases, and like all autoimmune disorders, occurs more frequently in women. Most patients with Hashimoto's thyroiditis have thyroid enlargement (goiter). Another, less common type of primary hypothyroidism is called autoimmune atrophic thyroiditis. In this disorder, TSH-blocking antibodies block the effect of TSH on the thyroid, leading to an atrophic gland.

Other common causes of primary hypothyroidism include thyroidectomy (e.g., for thyroid cancer) and ^{131}I ablation for hyperthyroidism. Iodine deficiency is rare in the United States but is still a common cause of hypothyroidism in underdeveloped countries. There are many drugs (e.g., lithium) that can also cause hypothyroidism.

In primary hypothyroidism, the thyroid fails to produce enough thyroid hormone, leading to low T4 and T3 levels. Because the pituitary is still intact, TSH levels rise. The elevated TSH level is the most sensitive indicator of hypothyroidism.

Too little thyroid hormone results in a sluggish individual with decreased energy. He or she often feels cold, complains of dry skin, muscle cramps, slowed mentation and speech, irregular menses (women), and constipation. Patients are able to perform normal activities in many cases. Obesity is not a result of hypothyroidism, contrary to the beliefs of many people. Most adults adapt to hypothyroidism quite well, and the symptoms abate after therapy. In cases of severe hypothyroidism, a condition called myxedema coma results, and may cause death.

Hypothyroidism in young children has more serious consequences. Cretinism is a condition caused by hypothyroidism in very young children and results in short stature and mental retardation. This is really the only endocrine syndrome that may result in mental retardation. Fortunately, this is extremely rare today, because mandatory testing for hypothyroidism in neonates is required in the United States and most developed countries.

Luckily, hypothyroidism is easily and inexpensively treated. In the old days, the patients had to undergo injections of thyroid hormone since oral preparations were not available. Later it was discovered that T4 is well absorbed orally. T4 is a small molecule that easily survives the cooking process, so one initial oral treatment of hypothyroidism was to give the patient cooked animal thyroid glands (sounds tasty). The next step was to make purer preparations from porcine and bovine thyroid glands, which are still available today. The preferred treatment today is synthetic levothyroxine, given once per day. Organic molecules come in both "right-handed" (dextro-) and "left-handed" (levo-) forms—almost all such molecules found in living organisms are the left-handed variety. Right-handed molecules (e.g., dextrothyroxine) are not useable by the body. The synthetic T4 is metabolized to T3 in the bloodstream, just like T4 secreted from the thyroid. Synthetic T4 is preferred to preparations made from animal thyroid glands, because it can be made with greater purity. We could give T3, but this is not ideal because its short half-life requires several doses per day. Treatment of primary hypothyroidism is monitored with routine TSH tests. With adequate treatment, the TSH returns to normal. In secondary hypothyroidism, the hormone levels themselves must be measured, since TSH secretion is already deficient.

Are there any circumstances in which hypothyroidism might actually be beneficial? For patients with severe coronary artery disease, hypothyroidism may be protective. The lowered basal metabolic rate protects the heart from working too hard. To this day there are actually three "approved" indications for therapeutic use of radioiodine (^{131}I). You may be aware of two (hyperthyroidism and thyroid carcinoma), but the third is an archaic one of historical significance: treatment of unstable angina. Remember, 40 or 50 years ago there was no such thing as coronary artery bypass grafting, angioplasty, or other interventional procedures for cardiac patients, nor was medical therapy very advanced (nitroglycerin was the mainstay of therapy). There just wasn't much available to help these folks with bad heart disease. For selected persons with coronary disease, hypothyroidism was actually induced by giving ^{131}I, which helped prolong their lives.

Treatment of hypothyroidism today in persons with coronary disease can still be risky business. Overzealous replacement can precipitate angina or even a myocardial infarction. It is best to try and correct underlying problems, if possible, before starting therapy.

HYPERTHYROIDISM AND THYROTOXICOSIS

This is the opposite of hypothyroidism, and is caused by thyroid hormone levels that are too high. The terms hyperthyroidism and thyrotoxicosis actually mean two different things. Thyrotoxicosis refers to excess thyroid hormone from any source (inside or outside the body), while hyperthyroidism refers to increased thyroid hormone levels from the body's own thyroid only. For simplicity, we will use these terms interchangeably. Thyrotoxicosis results in an "accelerated," hyperkinetic individual. Symptoms include weight loss, tachycardia (fast heart rate), increased appetite, tremors, inability to tolerate heat, and diarrhea. At first glance, it might seem beneficial to have all this excess energy and be able to do things much more quickly. Although thought processes are indeed faster, thyrotoxic persons often make mental errors. An analogy in the computer world is the "overclocking" of a computer microprocessor. Computer users discovered that running a microprocessor at a higher speed resulted in a faster computer without having to pay for a more expensive chip. For example, many users ran their 300 MHz processors at 450 MHz. The computers indeed were faster, but computational errors and early microprocessor breakdown were the occasional penalties. Another potentially desirable effect of thyrotoxicosis is the ability to lose weight easily. Many patients with thyrotoxicosis find that they can eat anything they want and still keep their weight down. At closer inspection, however, this is not such a good thing. The excess thyroid hormone does not only burn off fat but also bone and muscle. Indeed, patients with thyrotoxicosis often have significant muscle weakness and even develop osteoporosis because of the increased bone breakdown. It is much better for the patient to be a little bit overweight and have normal thyroid hormone levels than be thin and hyperthyroid.

We may define hyperthyroidism as either primary or secondary. Primary refers to the thyroid itself producing too much thyroid hormone without help from the pituitary gland. In primary hyperthyroidism, therefore, TSH levels are low since the pituitary wants nothing to do with this process. T4 and T3 levels are, of course, elevated. Almost all hyperthyroidism is primary in nature and we will focus on this. Secondary hyperthyroidism results from excessive production of TSH, and as we will discuss later, this is extremely uncommon.

Three basic mechanisms can result in thyrotoxicosis with low TSH. First, the thyroid may synthesize too much thyroid hormone. Second, the thyroid can "leak" large amounts of hormone that has already been made and is in storage (remember that the colloid is a vast reservoir of stored thyroid hormone). Lastly, a person can ingest too much thyroid hormone (overmedication).

THYROID HORMONE OVERPRODUCTION

The most common cause of thyroid hormone overproduction is called Graves' disease, another autoimmune endocrine disease. Unlike most autoimmune diseases (which cause gland hypofunction), Graves' disease results in hyperfunction. An antibody that binds to the thyroid and mimics TSH (an "imposter" TSH) causes this. Although TSH levels are low, the thyroid thinks it is being stimulated (because of the imposter TSH).

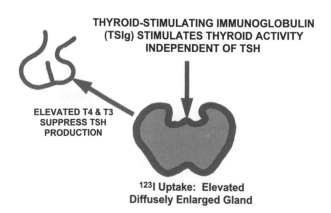

THYROID-STIMULATING IMMUNOGLOBULIN (TSIg) STIMULATES THYROID ACTIVITY INDEPENDENT OF TSH

ELEVATED T4 & T3 SUPPRESS TSH PRODUCTION

123I Uptake: Elevated Diffusely Enlarged Gland

Thyroid nodules also may "go haywire" and make too much thyroid hormone, resulting in hyperthyroidism. A single nodule may be the culprit (toxic nodule), or multiple nodules may be responsible (toxic multinodular goiter). "Goiter" is a generic term for thyroid enlargement. The whole thyroid may be enlarged (diffuse goiter), or be nodular (nodular goiter). These are like renegade players who follow plays called by the quarterback (the pituitary gland). Even though TSH levels are low, they continue misbehaving.

A radioiodine uptake and scan is often performed to verify this type of hyperthyroidism. Those with Graves' disease have a diffusely increased uptake (diffuse toxic goiter), whereas those with hyperfunctioning nodules have scans with a nodular pattern (with suppression of the neighboring normal thyroid tissue, which is "turned off" because of low TSH).

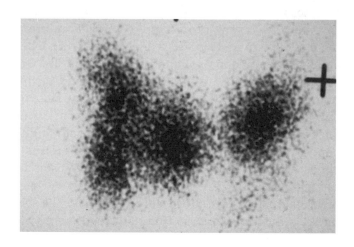

The treatment of this type of hyperthyroidism aims to get the thyroid to "slow down." There are three ways to accomplish this. This first is to surgically remove the thyroid. This is not always advised because of the small risk of damaging other delicate structures in the neck. Another way is to give medications that hinder thyroid hormone synthesis. The two antithyroid medications that accomplish this are propylthiouracil (PTU) and methimazole. These medications are similar to compounds (thioureas) found in cabbage and brussels sprouts, and taste bitter to many people. (The ability to taste thioureas was one of the earliest examples of classical Mendelian inheritance.) These drugs generally only work as long as the patient is taking them, although some patients may spontaneously go into remission. Some experts have proposed immune-modifying effects of these drugs.

Another type of medication we often give patients with hyperthyroidism is the β-blocker. Remember that one of the effects of thyroid hormone is to stimulate the sympathetic nervous system (resulting in tremors and tachycardia). β-blockers (e.g., propranolol, metoprolol) decrease the systemic effects of thyroid hormones and alleviate symptoms very quickly. Since they block the adrenergic effects of thyroid hormones and therefore are not dependent on the etiology of hyperthyroidism, they are useful for all forms of hyperthyroidism. They do not, obviously, treat the cause of hyperthyroidism.

The third method of treating this type of hyperthyroidism is to employ radioactive iodine (^{131}I). Treatment results in destruction of thyroid tissue and restoration of normal thyroid (euthyroid) hormone levels. Often, the radioactive iodine does too much damage, resulting in permanent hypothyroidism. Fortunately, this is easily and inexpensively treated. You might ask why we cannot give just enough radioactive iodine to render the patient euthyroid. In theory, this would be a good idea—in practice, however, this often does not work. If we give too little radioactive iodine, the patient often ends up relapsing, requiring a second or third treatment.

Some other problems may occur in patients with Graves' disease. The antibodies, in addition to the thyroid, may stimulate other tissues. The most common associated condition is exophthalmos, which causes protrusion of the eyes (proptosis) and enlargement of the eye muscles. This condition may result in impaired eye movement and loss of visual acuity. Permanent visual impairment may result in severe cases. Fortunately, most patients with proptosis do not go on to develop significant eye problems. Patients with Graves' disease should always see an eye specialist on a routine basis.

Because exophthalmos is caused by antibodies and not elevated thyroid hormone levels, treatment of hyperthyroidism does not necessarily improve eye disease in patients with Graves' disease. The antibodies are unaffected by treating the thyroid problem with any of the three methods mentioned above. Treatment of exophthalmos includes orbital radiation, extraocular muscle surgery, orbital decompression (to give the eye more room), and corticosteroids (which decrease inflammation).

A much less common condition occurring in patients with Graves' disease is pretibial myxedema, which results in pebbly orange skin on the shin areas. This is usually a minor problem and does not cause significant disability in most cases.

RELEASE OF PREFORMED THYROID HORMONE

The thyroid is like a big "water tank" with vast stores of thyroid hormone, contained in the proteinaceous colloid. This is unlike most endocrine glands that do not have large stores of their hormones. The stores of thyroid hormone are often enough to last for several weeks. Thus, if some mechanism irritates the thyroid so that hormone can "leak out," hyperthyroidism results. This is obviously a different mechanism than thyroid hormone overproduction.

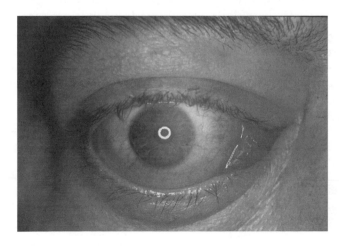

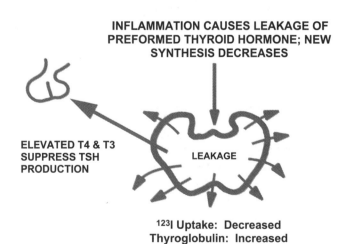

INFLAMMATION CAUSES LEAKAGE OF PREFORMED THYROID HORMONE; NEW SYNTHESIS DECREASES

ELEVATED T4 & T3 SUPPRESS TSH PRODUCTION

LEAKAGE

^{123}I Uptake: Decreased
Thyroglobulin: Increased

This type of thyroid "irritation" is called subacute thyroiditis. It is often accompanied by pain in the thyroid gland. A variant, occurring in many postpartum women, is called postpartum thyroiditis.

Leakage of stored thyroid hormone results in increased T4 and T3 levels, and symptoms of hyperthyroidism. Since new thyroid hormone is not being produced, the uptake of the radioiodine is diminished. This results in the seemingly confusing association of low radioiodine uptake and hyperthyroidism. When you think about the physiology, however, it makes sense. In contrast, in cases of hyperthyroidism due to thyroid hormone overproduction, the thyroid uptake is elevated.

We can't do a whole lot about thyroid hormone that has already been synthesized. Antithyroid drugs such as propylthiouracil have no effect, since no new hormone is being made. Radioiodine therapy also would be useless, since uptake is low and the thyroid would not accumulate a significant amount of ^{131}I. Removing the thyroid surgically is not a good idea, since this procedure might irritate the thyroid even more and release more stored hormone into the circulation. β-blockers do help with the symptoms and are used routinely. Nonsteroidal anti-inflammatory agents (e.g., ibuprofen) or corticosteroids decrease inflammation and may be useful to decrease the leakage.

Fortunately, like a water tank that springs a leak, there is only a finite amount of substance inside, which will eventually run out. Thyroid hormone levels in time will actually drop below normal, producing a temporary state of hypothyroidism. It may take several weeks for the thyroid to rebuild its stores, at which time the patient is again euthyroid. Rarely, the inflammation is so severe that the thyroid cannot regenerate completely, resulting in permanent hypothyroidism. This is easily treated with daily thyroxine replacement.

EXOGENOUS INGESTION OF THYROID HORMONE

Another cause of thyrotoxicosis with low radioiodine uptake occurs in those who take too much thyroid hormone because the dosage of thyroxine is too high. It can also occur in people who illicitly take thyroid hormone, often in an effort to lose weight. This most commonly occurs in health care providers with access to readily available thyroid hormone.

Another interesting example of this type of thyrotoxicosis occurred many years ago. Remember that an early therapy for hypothyroidism was the ingestion of animal thyroid glands. It appears that in one part of the country, a batch of hamburger was made from beef in which the thyroid glands had not been removed. The thyroid glands were ground up with hamburger resulting in large amounts of T4. The T4 survived cooking and resulted in thyrotoxicosis in many patients. This phenomenon was appropriately termed "hamburger thyrotoxicosis."

It is important to distinguish this type of thyrotoxicosis from another type that presents with a low radioiodine uptake (subacute thyroiditis). Remember how thyroxine is stored in the colloid, attached to a protein called thyroglobulin (Tg). With thyroiditis and release of thyroid hormone, the thyroglobulin is released into the bloodstream too, resulting in an increased Tg level. Those who take too much hormone have low Tg levels, since Tg is not contained in the thyroxine tablet.

SECONDARY HYPERTHYROIDISM

As we discussed above, secondary hyperthyroidism is quite rare. TSH-secreting pituitary tumors produce elevated TSH and T4 levels. This condition is readily distinguished from primary hyperthyroidism by the increased TSH levels. Treatment includes medication (octreotide) and/or surgical resection. Another cause of secondary hyperthyroidism is pituitary thyroid hormone resistance, in which the pituitary is resistant to levels of T4 and T3 in the circulation. Since TSH does not suppress normally, it continues stimulating the thyroid and hyperthyroidism may result.

SEVERE THYROTOXICOSIS: THYROID STORM

Thyroid storm is a condition caused by severe thyrotoxicosis. Graves' disease is the typical cause, and other forms of hyperthyroidism only rarely result in symptoms of this degree. These persons present with fever, confusion, severe tachycardia, and may suffer cardiovascular collapse. The mortality rate is high if untreated. Treatment includes β-blockers and antithyroid drugs.

THYROID NODULES

A goiter is a generic term for any thyroid enlargement. Goiters may be diffuse as in Graves' disease, or nodular. Nodular goiters are common, especially in women. A patient may have either a single (solitary) nodule, or multiple nodules (multinodular goiter). They are usually euthyroid, although hypo- or hyperthyroidism may also be associated with thyroid nodules. The main concern is whether the nodule is benign or malignant.

Fortunately, most thyroid nodules are benign, especially those that have remained unchanged for years. Those that are rapidly growing are more likely to be malignant. In the glorious "atomic age" of the 1950s, doctors gave radiation treatments for a variety of benign conditions ranging from acne to enlarged tonsils. We know now that these radiation treatments resulted in a small increase in the incidence of thyroid cancer; therefore, a careful history must be obtained from each patient.

How do we evaluate nodules? A costly way is to perform a radionuclide thyroid scan. A nodule may not concentrate radioiodine as well as surrounding thyroid tissue, leading to a "punched out" or "cold" nodule appearance on the scan. If it concentrates radioiodine as well, it cannot be distinguished from normal thyroid and is called "warm." A hyperfunctioning nodule ("hot nodule") suppresses the surrounding thyroid tissue.

Unfortunately, this information is really not very useful to us. It is a common belief that cold nodules are usually malignant, but this is not true. They are somewhat more likely to be malignant than hot nodules, but most cold nodules (at least 80%) are benign. Some also erroneously think that hot nodules cannot be cancerous, but alas, carcinoma can arise in such nodules. As a result, it turns out that a thyroid scan is not very useful in evaluating euthyroid patients with thyroid nodules.

A better way of delineating anatomy is to perform a thyroid ultrasound. This can demonstrate the depth of a nodule (whereas a radionuclide scan only yields a poor quality, two-dimensional frontal picture). Cystic (fluid-filled) nodules are less likely to be malignant than solid ones, but this maxim does not always hold true. If you really want to know the nature and size of the nodules, an ultrasound is the way to go.

We haven't yet mentioned a really good way to distinguish benign from malignant nodules. Since thyroid nodules are so common, we need a better test. The best way is to actually look at thyroid cells under a microscope, by a procedure called fine needle aspiration. This is done with a very small needle, and causes minimal discomfort to the patient. Ultrasound may be used to guide the needle with nodules that are difficult to feel. The sensitivity (ability of the test to detect cancer) is about 95% in the hands of a skilled clinician. If two biopsies are done, this figure approaches 99%.

If the nodule is malignant, it should obviously be removed. If benign, no treatment is necessary. Some seemingly benign tumors (e.g., follicular adenomas) should be removed because they may harbor occult cancerous cells. Suppression with thyroxine has been employed in the past, but recent studies show that this treatment is of little benefit to most patients. Those that are cosmetically disfiguring may be removed. Others are simply followed with regular examinations.

DIFFERENTIATED (EPITHELIAL) THYROID CARCINOMA

The words "carcinoma" and cancer sound ominous. Fortunately, the most common types of thyroid cancer grow very slowly and rarely cause death. These are the epithelial thyroid cancers, papillary and follicular cancer, and account for 95% of those with thyroid cancer. They are called epithelial thyroid cancers because they arise from follicular epithelium and not from other cells within the thyroid. Papillary is the most common. No one wants to have cancer, but if you had to pick a cancer to have, this is the type to get. Most patients have lesions confined to the thyroid. Very, very rarely, metastases and death occur, usually many years after diagnosis and treatment. Follicular cancer is a bit more aggressive than papillary, but most patients do well.

The cornerstone of treatment of epithelial thyroid cancers is removal of the thyroid. The majority of patients are cured by this treatment alone. After the thyroid has been completely removed by the surgeon, all the cancer is usually gone. The method by which we follow this type of cancer, however, necessitates another type of treatment. We follow thyroid cancer by two means: (a) radioiodine scanning, or (b) serum thyroglobulin (Tg) levels. The scan will not work properly, however, until every last bit of the thyroid is gone. If there is even a microscopic amount of normal thyroid left (called "remnants"), it will take up the tracer rather than the possible tumor, and the scan will be fruitless. We measure Tg, since it is a marker of thyroid epithelial tissue—if levels go up it means the cancer could be coming back. However, the thyroid remnant makes Tg too, and we can't distinguish Tg of normal thyroid epithelial origin from that of cancer tissue origin.

Therefore, we must get rid of these small remnants in order to see a tumor in the patient's body or rely on serum Tg levels. This is easily done with a high-dose ^{131}I treatment, which basically burns up the small remaining pieces. Only after these are gone can we do a reliable scan to look for metastases (which hopefully are not there). This therapy is called a "remnant ablation." This is the same type of radioiodine used for hyperthyroidism, but is given in a higher dose.

The treatment itself is very simple. It involves swallowing a radioactive iodine capsule, similar to the thyroid scan. It is painless and does not involve intravenous lines or injections. Radioactive iodine usually does not cause side effects, and the radiation dose to the rest of the patient's body is quite small. Patients do not experience hair loss, nausea, or vomiting which can occur with other types of cancer therapy. Occasionally there is some tenderness in the neck area (radiation thyroiditis). They also might experience an unusual taste in their mouths or swelling of the salivary glands, which usually only lasts a few days.

Before the thyroid cancer survey, all thyroid hormone has to be out of the patient's system. This is because thyroid cancer cells are relatively insensitive to radioiodine, and high TSH levels must be present to stimulate cancer cells, if present, to take up the isotope. Can you think of a simple way to cause elevated TSH levels in a patient without a thyroid? The obvious method is to induce hypothyroidism by taking the patient off his or her thyroid hormone. The patient must discontinue thyroxine for several weeks for this to occur. Understandably, this causes patients to develop significant symptoms of hypothyroidism and feel very poorly.

Since the only reason to discontinue the thyroid hormone is to achieve high TSH levels, you might ask why we can't just give TSH to the patients to alleviate their discomfort. In the past, this was impossible because TSH was not available. Today, however, synthetic human TSH is readily available, and can be given to patients via an injection before the scan, eliminating the need to stop thyroid hormone in many patients.

A follow-up scan may be done in a year or two. Serum thyroglobulin (Tg) levels are also monitored, and hopefully will be low. If a scan shows metastases or Tg levels rise, a repeat high-dose radioiodine therapy may be necessary.

MEDULLARY AND ANAPLASTIC THYROID CARCINOMA

Medullary thyroid carcinoma (MTC) is a less common type of thyroid cancer arising in the parafollicular (C) cells of the thyroid, which manufacture the hormone calcitonin. This is a much more aggressive form of thyroid cancer, and those with widespread metastases have a poor prognosis. This type of tumor does not make thyroglobulin and does not concentrate radioiodine well, so treatment with the latter is usually ineffective. Serum calcitonin levels are usually elevated, and useful to follow as a marker of tumor burden. Treatment with external radiation therapy and/or chemotherapy may offer palliative benefit in those with severe disease.

Anaplastic carcinoma is by far the most aggressive thyroid cancer, and one of the most lethal of all cancers. It presents as rapid thyroid enlargement, often over a matter of days. There is no effective treatment, and most patients die within weeks to months. This type of tumor is not responsive to radioactive iodine.

4 ADRENAL GLAND

REVIEW

In the previous lecture we learned about our first major endocrine system controlled by the hypothalamus and pituitary—the thyroid gland. This gland is of paramount importance because of the thyroid's effects on the other organ systems.

T4 is the major thyroid hormone secreted by the thyroid. It is made up of two modified tyrosine molecules with four iodine atoms attached. T3 is the most potent thyroid hormone and is primarily made by the peripheral conversion of T4 in the peripheral circulation by a deiodinase. The trophic hormone for T4 production is the pituitary hormone TSH. Under the influence of TSH, iodine is organified (attached to the thyronine molecules) and stored within the functional unit of the thyroid (follicle) in colloid attached to a protein called thyroglobulin. When needed, T4 is secreted from the colloid into the bloodstream.

Common measurements of thyroid function include the iodothyronines T4 and T3, as well as pituitary TSH. The thyroid scan is a common nuclear medicine study. This is an image of the thyroid taken after administration of radioactive iodine. A thyroid uptake is the fractional accumulation of radioactive iodine after a set period of time. ^{123}I is most commonly used for imaging; ^{131}I is used for destroying thyroid tissue (e.g., hyperthyroidism and thyroid cancer).

Hypothyroidism is one of the most common endocrine diseases. The most common cause is the autoimmune disorder Hashimoto's thyroiditis. In primary hypothyroidism, TSH levels rise in an effort to stimulate the thyroid. The elevated TSH level, therefore, is the most sensitive indicator of hypothyroidism. Symptoms of hypothyroidism include cold intolerance, dry skin, muscle cramps, slowed mentation, irregular menses in women, and constipation. Untreated hypothyroidism in children results in a serious condition called cretinism. Fortunately, hypothyroidism is inexpensively and easily treated with thyroid hormone. Synthetic thyroxine is the treatment of choice.

Hyperthyroidism, or thyrotoxicosis, is the condition of thyroid hormone excess and has a variety of causes. The first type results from production of too much thyroid hormone. The most common cause is Graves' disease, which also is an autoimmune disease. It is unique in that it is one of the few autoimmune diseases that results in endocrine excess. Thyroid nodules that produce too much thyroid hormone (toxic adenoma) are another common cause of thyroid hormone overproduction. Treatment of this type of hyperthyroidism includes antithyroid medication, radioactive iodine therapy, or surgery.

Hyperthyroidism may also be caused by leakage of preformed thyroid hormone. This is illustrated by destructive thyroiditis, in which irritation of the thyroid leads to spillage of preformed hormone. In contrast to thyroid hormone overproduction, the thyroid uptake in this type of hyperthyroidism is decreased. This type of hyperthyroidism normally resolves on its own. Another cause of hyperthyroidism is the ingestion of too much thyroid hormone. This usually occurs in individuals who are trying to lose weight or have psychiatric problems.

Thyroid nodules are quite common, especially in women. Most often they are benign. Radionuclide thyroid scans are generally a poor choice for evaluating thyroid nodules, since they do not reliably distinguish benign from malignant lesions. The best way to distinguish a benign from a malignant thyroid nodule is to perform a fine needle aspiration biopsy.

Thyroid carcinomas may be divided into two types: carcinomas arising from epithelial tissue (papillary and follicular carcinoma), and the non-epithelial varieties (medullary and anaplastic carcinoma). Epithelial thyroid carcinomas are treated by surgical excision and radioactive iodine therapy. The others types of thyroid cancer do not respond to radioactive iodine, and surgery is the mainstay of therapy.

THE ADRENAL GLANDS

In this lecture we will study the adrenal glands, which are often called the "fight or flight" glands because they secrete hormones that are necessary for homeostasis under physical stress. In our football team analogy, they are like the halfback or wide receiver who is capable of blocking, but also capable of accelerating many times to break the big play. The adrenals are paired glands that lie in the retroperitoneal cavity above the kidneys. They have two functional parts—most of the adrenal consists of the outer cortex, with the remainder being the inner medulla.

The adrenal cortex contains three layers, or zones, and makes steroid hormones, which are derived from cholesterol. The only other organs that synthesize steroids are the gonads (ovaries and testes), which make sex steroids. The outermost cortical layer, called the zona glomerulosa, is responsible for synthesizing steroids that help us retain salt and water; hence this layer's principal steroid, aldosterone, is called a mineralocorticoid. This hormone is necessary for life.

The thickest or middle layer, the zona fasciculata, makes another life-sustaining group of hormones, the glucocorticoids. As the name implies, these compounds are important in helping the body maintain adequate glucose (energy) levels. The major glucocorticoid is cortisol (hydrocortisone).

The thinnest cortical layer is the innermost (the zona fasciculata), which provides adrenal androgen secretion in both men and women. Most testosterone in the male originates from the testes, however. These hormones are not necessary to sustain life.

The inner medulla is the site of catecholamine synthesis. The catecholamine hormones (e.g., epinephrine) are important during stressful physiologic situations.

All steroids are synthesized from cholesterol. For cholesterol to be useful, it must be transported to the mitochondria by StAR (steroidogenic acute regulatory protein). In the mitochondrion, cholesterol is converted to pregnenolone by cholesterol side-chain cleavage enzyme. All steroids of the cortex are made from pregnenolone by a variety of different enzymes (see the following figure). Most of these are in the family of cytochrome P450 oxygenases. Drugs that inhibit enzymes in the P450 system (e.g., ketoconazole) may inhibit steroid synthesis.

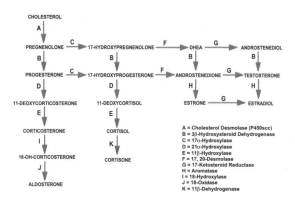

Let's discuss the glucocorticoids first. Although all adrenal steroids are made in the cortex, glucocorticoids are sometimes called corticosteroids because of their great importance. Their name is derived from their ability to increase glucose concentrations via increased gluconeogenesis and decreased glucose uptake. They are therefore activated when the body is in a hungry state or otherwise needs energy. Life is not possible without normal amounts of these hormones. In excess amounts, they inhibit protein synthesis and promote protein breakdown, since they are meant to help the body obtain energy.

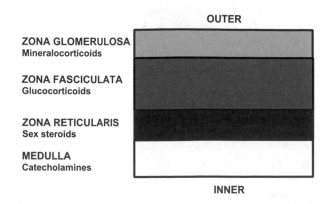

	OUTER
ZONA GLOMERULOSA Mineralocorticoids	
ZONA FASCICULATA Glucocorticoids	
ZONA RETICULARIS Sex steroids	
MEDULLA Catecholamines	
	INNER

Cortisol (hydrocortisone)

Cortisone

Aldosterone

Like most endocrine organs, the zona fasciculata is under control of a feedback loop. It and the zona reticularis—site of male hormone (androgen) synthesis—is essentially a separate organ from the aldosterone-synthesizing glomerulosa, and are under different control. The stimulus for the zona fasciculata is the anterior pituitary hormone ACTH (adrenocorticotropic hormone, corticotropin). Under stimulation by ACTH, this layer increases production of its hormone. Minutes after ACTH levels increase, cortisol levels increase. This phenomenon can be observed by measuring serum cortisol levels before and after ACTH infusion.

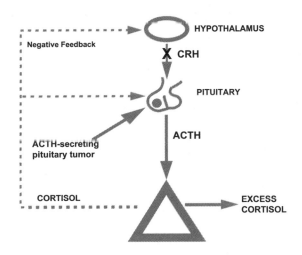

After cortisol levels reach a certain plateau, it tells the pituitary that there is enough and to slow down ACTH production. Under times of stress (e.g., surgery, sepsis, or even strenuous exercise), ACTH levels increase to produce more cortisol (to provide the body with more energy). The body can produce as much as ten times the normal amount of cortisol, if necessary. One of the biggest physiological stresses of all is pregnancy.

CORTISOL EXCESS: CUSHING'S SYNDROME

Normally, this all works quite well and cortisol levels remain normal. Occasionally, something goes wrong with the body and too much cortisol is produced. This is called Cushing's syndrome (named after Harvey Cushing, a famous neurosurgeon), and may have several different causes.

Let's think of the ways that the body could produce too much cortisol. If there is too much ACTH, the cortex would make too much cortisol. Cushing's disease is a subtype of Cushing's syndrome caused by an ACTH-secreting pituitary tumor. This is the most common cause of endogenous CS (i.e., the source of cortisol originates within the body).

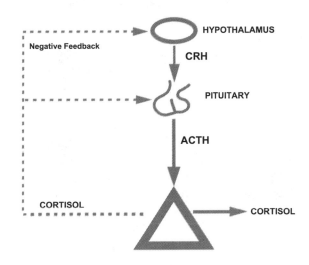

There are other tumors that can make ACTH also. These include neuroendocrine tumors such as small (oat) cell lung carcinoma, which can also manufacture other neuroendocrine peptides. Since the source of ACTH is outside its native source (the pituitary), this syndrome is called "ectopic" (paraneoplastic or "out of place") ACTH syndrome. This is the second most common cause of endogenous CS. In these causes of CS, the ACTH level is elevated, often hundreds to thousands of times normal in ectopic ACTH syndrome, which tends to be much more aggressive than Cushing's disease.

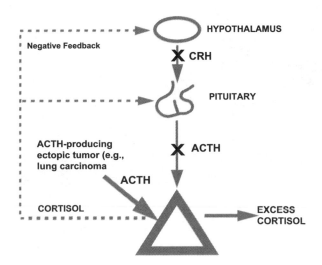

CS may also occur if the adrenal goes haywire and makes too much cortisol on its own, without regulation by ACTH. This type occurs with tumors that do not respond to normal feedback. These may be benign tumors (adenomas), or malignant (adrenocortical carcinomas). The latter tend to be very aggressive and are often fatal. Since the pituitary works normally, ACTH levels are "shut off" (low).

The most common cause of CS is exogenous (i.e., the source of the steroid is outside the body). Synthetic glucocorticoids are used for many conditions, including chronic rheumatologic and pulmonary disease, and those receiving immunosuppression for organ transplants. These persons must receive very high doses of steroids to suppress their disease or prevent organ rejection. Exogenous CS is usually obvious, since it is known to the health care provider that the person is on steroids. Since the pituitary sees too much cortisol, ACTH levels are low.

The clinical features of CS are due to the deleterious effects of cortisol excess. Skin strength is diminished, and easy bruising and pigmented striae (stretch marks) are common. Cortisol excess destroys muscle mass, so these people tend to be very weak, especially in the proximal limb muscles. It is common for even a young person with CS to be unable to do a deep knee bend without help. Osteoporosis is common, and a presenting complaint may be a pathologic fracture. They may develop central obesity and a characteristic fat deposition in the cervical area ("buffalo hump"). A round "moon face" is common.

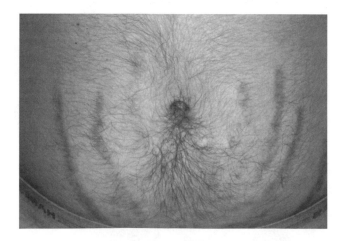

There are several ways to screen a patient for CS. Because of the periodic nature of ACTH and hence cortisol secretion, random values are often of little value. A tried-and-true screening test is the measurement of urine cortisol excretion over a 24-hour period. A normal value rules against CS, while an elevated level warrants further investigation. Another screening test is the dexamethasone suppression test. This test exploits the ability of an administered synthetic glucocorticoid (dexamethasone) to suppress ACTH and cortisol secretion in the normal individual. If we give dexamethasone to a normal person in the evening, the cortisol level should drop very low by the next morning, because of physiologic suppression of ACTH production. In the person with CS, the level does not drop. Either the ACTH level does not fall low enough (in the ACTH-dependent forms, Cushing's disease and ectopic ACTH), or the rampant adrenal continues to work on its own (adrenal tumors). This is just a screening test, and like the 24-hour urine cortisol test, a confirmatory test is needed.

The confirmatory test for CS is another type of DST, the low-dose test. In this test, .05 mg dexamethasone is given every 6 hours for 2 days, and serum cortisol and urine cortisol levels are measured. In normal persons, the levels suppress and in those with CS, they do not.

A more recent test is the measurement of salivary cortisol levels. Here, the patient places small cotton plugs in the mouth, and cortisol levels are measured in the evening. This test has shown much promise and may replace some of the cumbersome dexamethasone suppression tests, which sometimes yield confusing results.

Once CS is confirmed, how do we isolate the cause? The ACTH level is valuable here. If elevated, CS cannot be caused by adrenal tumors, since the high cortisol levels tell the HPA (hypothalamic-pituitary axis) to shut off. If elevated, we are then left with CD versus ectopic ACTH. A pituitary MRI may show a tumor, which suggests CD. A large lung tumor suggests ectopic ACTH syndrome. In cases where these studies are equivocal, a technique called petrosal sinus sampling is done. Here, ACTH is actually measured from the petrosal sinuses (which drain the pituitary), and compared to ACTH in the peripheral blood. Pituitary ACTH levels higher than peripheral levels suggest CD. If not, ectopic ACTH syndrome is suggested. If the ACTH level is low, adrenal computed tomography (CT) or MRI may isolate the tumor.

The cause of CS is then treated. For Cushing's disease, the pituitary tumor is removed. With small tumors, this probably will leave normal residual pituitary function. With large tumors, the pituitary may be damaged, requiring hormone replacement. Ectopic ACTH syndrome is often not curable, because of the aggressive nature of many tumors. The tumor (e.g., lung cancer) is treated by whatever means necessary, and may be palliative. Drugs that slow down adrenal steroid synthesis (e.g., ketoconazole) may be considered.

Adrenal tumors should be surgically removed, since the body can function quite well with only one adrenal gland. Adrenocortical cancers are much more aggressive and may not be curable. Metastases are frequent and often fatal. Reducing the dosage of administered glucocorticoid to the lowest possible level can minimize iatrogenic CS.

ADRENOCORTICAL INSUFFICIENCY: ADDISON'S DISEASE

Each endocrine organ has a deficiency syndrome as well as a hormonal excess syndrome. Since the adrenal cortex is necessary for life, it would stand to reason that adrenal insufficiency could cause many problems. Like all deficiency syndromes, adrenal insufficiency (AI) may be primary or secondary. Primary AI occurs when the adrenal gland itself is damaged. Secondary AI occurs if the cortex has atrophied because of insufficient ACTH.

Primary AI is also called Addison's disease, named after Thomas Addison, who described the condition in 1849. Like most endocrine deficiency syndromes, the most common cause is autoimmune. Other causes include tuberculosis, congenital adrenal enzyme defects, fungal infection (histoplasmosis), infiltrative diseases (hemochromatosis), and metastatic cancer.

Since cortisol is a stress hormone, it stands to reason that those with AI don't have a lot of energy. Indeed, these persons are frequently weak, anorexic, hypoglycemic, and depressed. As a young man, President John F. Kennedy developed weakness, weight loss, and hyperpigmentation, and he finally was diagnosed as having Addison's disease.

In primary endocrine deficiency disorders, the trophic hormone always rises in a futile effort to get the gland working. In this case, ACTH rises, often to hundreds of times above normal. An interesting property of ACTH is its similarity to the hormone melanocyte-stimulating hormone (α-MSH), which isn't very important in humans. This hormone is important in many lower vertebrates (e.g., reptiles and amphibians) who change color to blend with their environment and escape predators. In humans, melanocytes are responsible for moles, freckles, and suntan. The very high ACTH levels in Addison's disease act like MSH and cause increased melanin deposition and hyperpigmentation in the skin. (MSH, however, has no ACTH-like activity.) Indeed, those with Addison's disease often look like they just came in from weeks in the Florida sun. In fact, early on in the disease, some patients are actually pleased because they lose weight and have a nice suntan, without any effort! This is not a good way to get a tan, though. They eventually become ill and seek medical treatment.

You might ask if those with Cushing's disease or ectopic ACTH syndrome develop hyperpigmentation. Those with Cushing's disease usually do not have sufficient ACTH to develop this problem, but levels are frequently high enough in ectopic ACTH syndrome to cause it.

There are some common laboratory abnormalities in those with Addison's disease. Since cortisol is important for glucose metabolism, hypoglycemia may be seen. Aldosterone is important in helping the body get rid of potassium and hold onto sodium, and hyperkalemia and hyponatremia are often seen. Cortisol is also important in helping the body hold onto sodium. Patients may be dehydrated, so serum blood urea nitrogen (BUN) and creatinine may be elevated.

Patients may go for years with mild disease and only minor symptoms. Often, it is suspected because the person fails to recover from minor illnesses easily (e.g., viral infections). If subjected to enough stress, adrenal crisis or shock may result. This can happen if the previously undiagnosed AI sufferer is in an accident, undergoes surgery, or has a serious illness (e.g., myocardial infarction), which precipitates the adrenal crisis.

Fortunately, Addison's disease (primary adrenal insufficiency) is easily and inexpensively treated. Cortisone was isolated in 1949 (100 years after the original description of primary adrenal insufficiency by Addison) and was deemed a wonder drug. Patients with Addison's may receive an oral glucocorticoid, such as the naturally occurring hydrocortisone or cortisone. Alternatively, a synthetic glucocorticoid such as prednisone or dexamethasone can be used. The reason for the natural steroids is their intrinsic mineralocorticoid activity, and some patients do well on hydrocortisone alone. Others require addition of a synthetic mineralocorticoid such as fludrocortisone (aldosterone is degraded after oral administration). A patient with adrenal insufficiency must increase his or her steroid dose during severe stress (e.g., illness or surgery).

INBORN ERRORS OF CORTISOL BIOSYNTHESIS: CONGENITAL ADRENAL HYPERPLASIA

The congenital adrenal hyperplasias (CAH) are a group of autosomal recessive disorders of steroid biosynthesis. There are several different types, depending on the enzymatic block. The common element in each is that an end product is not made, leading to increase in ACTH and hence adrenal hyperplasia. The clinical findings seen depend on the enzyme defect and the precursor that accumulates. Problems seen include virilization (increased androgens and precursors), feminization (decreased androgens), adrenal insufficiency (decreased glucocorticoids), and/or hypertension (increased mineralocorticoid precursors). A vicious cycle is produced in which inadequate formation of an end product (e.g., cortisol) leads to increased ACTH and accumulation of precursors (e.g., androgen) since the desired product cannot be made adequately.

The most common type of CAH is 21-hydroxylase deficiency. In this disorder, the enzymatic block leads to inadequate aldosterone and cortisol production, and adrenal crisis and shock shortly after birth if untreated. Instead, androgenic precursors accumulate, resulting in virilization of girls, ambiguous genitalia, and female pseudohermaphrodism (male appearance in a genetic female). It is the most common cause of ambiguous genitalia in the female. In boys, it results in virilization at an early age, causing severe psychological and developmental problems. In both sexes, early excess of sex steroids results in precocious puberty, with an initial increase in growth velocity and eventual short stature due to early fusion of the epiphyseal plates (from androgen excess).

The goals of treatment are prevention of adrenal crisis and death, early recognition in the female so that she can be reared as the correct sex, and early treatment in both sexes to prevent precocious puberty and the resultant short adult stature and psychological problems.

All forms of CAH are treated by administering glucocorticoids (e.g., hydrocortisone), which decrease ACTH levels to normal and reduce synthesis of excess steroid precursors. Mineralocorticoids (fludrocortisone) may also be required in some patients.

MINERALOCORTICOIDS

Aldosterone is the primary mineralocorticoid and is produced by the zona glomerulosa layer of the adrenal cortex. The purpose of this hormone is helping the body to hold on to sodium and excrete potassium, hence the name "mineralocorticoid." Unlike the inner two layers, ACTH is not necessary for its proper secretion. Instead, it is under the regulation of the renin-angiotensin system, involving the kidneys and liver. The stimulus for aldosterone secretion begins in the kidney, which secretes the hormone renin in response to hypotension, decreased intravascular volume, increased serum osmolality, and hyperkalemia. Under the influence of renin, the hepatic peptide angiotensinogen is converted to angiotensin I. Another enzyme, angiotensin converting enzyme, converts angiotensin I to angiotensin II. Angiotensin II then stimulates the zona glomerulosa to make aldosterone. Aldosterone then does its thing, by helping the body retain salt and water and excrete potassium. Once these levels return to normal, the kidney stops making renin and all is well.

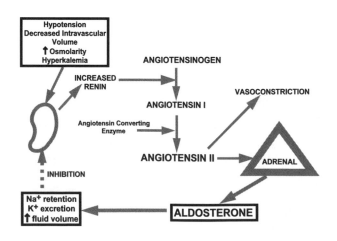

Those with secondary adrenal insufficiency (due to pituitary or hypothalamic disease) do not require a mineralocorticoid, since the aldosterone layer is not ACTH-dependent. The zona glomerulosa goes on making aldosterone just fine without ACTH.

HYPERALDOSTERONISM

HYPERALDOSTERONISM

Just as glucocorticoids may be secreted in excess, mineralocorticoid hypersecretion may also occur, leading to the clinical syndrome of hyperaldosteronism. Here, excess aldosterone results in potassium loss from the kidneys, low serum potassium levels (hypokalemia), and hypertension. It is suggested by the finding of spontaneous hypokalemia (i.e., not due to drugs such as diuretics) with elevated serum and/or urinary aldosterone levels. Primary hyperaldosteronism is due to autonomous hypersecretion from the adrenal itself, and is not dependent on the renin-angiotensin system; renin levels are therefore low. **Secondary hyperaldosteronism is due to a condition that elevates renin levels. Most commonly this is due to renovascular hypertension. It also may be caused by a renin-secreting tumor.**

Primary aldosteronism is typically due to a benign adrenal tumor (Conn's syndrome). In most of the other cases, the hyperaldosteronism is due to enlargement (hyperplasia) of both adrenal glands. **Hyperaldosteronism is rarely caused by adrenocortical carcinoma and congenital adrenal enzyme defects. Glucocorticoid-remediable aldosteronism (GRA) is an uncommon genetic cause of hyperaldosteronism, which results in aldosterone production by the ACTH-dependent zona fasciculata. Administration of small doses of glucocorticoid (e.g., dexamethasone) ameliorates the hypertension and other biochemical findings.**

Tumors causing hyperaldosteronism are typically excised. The remaining adrenal is adequate for the rest of the body's needs. Hypokalemia usually resolves, and the hypertension improves. Hyperaldosteronism due to bilateral hyperplasia ("idiopathic" hyperaldosteronism) is best treated with medication, since removal of both adrenal glands does not help the hypertension. Adrenocortical carcinoma typically carries a poor prognosis.

CARDIAC HORMONES AND SODIUM METABOLISM

CARDIAC HORMONES AND SODIUM METABOLISM

In addition to antidiuretic hormone and mineralocorticoids, there are other factors that influence sodium excretion. It was discovered long ago that distention of the atrium resulted in increased water excretion. Later it was discovered that a peptide hormone, atrial natriuretic peptide (ANP), is secreted by cardiac atrial cells. Volume overload causes atrial distention, resulting in release of ANP. ANP primarily affects the kidney, where it results in natriuresis, increased glomerular filtration rate, and decreased renin secretion. It also inhibits adrenal cortical aldosterone production.

RENOVASCULAR HYPERTENSION (RENAL ARTERY STENOSIS)

Renal artery stenosis is a relatively common condition and is often caused by atherosclerotic disease. These lesions result in stenosis and decreased blood flow to the kidneys. This fools the kidneys into thinking that blood pressure is low, and tricks them into producing more renin. This in turn produces more angiotensin II and aldosterone, resulting in hypertension (a form of "secondary" aldosteronism). **Despite the increased blood pressure, the kidneys still think that the blood pressure is low (due to the stenotic lesions). This vicious cycle results in hypertension.**

This type of hypertension should be considered in any person under age 25 or over 55 who develops hypertension. It may be corrected with angioplasty (inflating a balloon across the stenotic lesion) or by surgically correcting the stenotic artery.

RENOVASCULAR HYPERTENSION

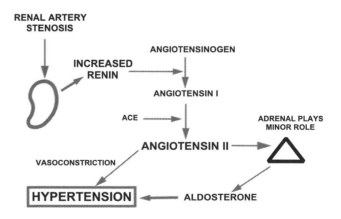

ADRENAL MEDULLA

For our purposes, we will consider the adrenal medulla a separate entity from the adrenal cortex. The medulla is responsible for secreting catecholamines (epinephrine, norepinephrine, and dopamine), which are made from the amino acid tyrosine. **The same types** of cells are also found in the central nervous system and in the sympathetic chain. The major catecholamine secreted by the medulla is epinephrine (adrenaline). Norepinephrine is more abundant in extramedullary tissues.

There are no well-defined trophic hormones for the adrenal medulla. The catecholamines tend to increase when the body experiences physical or mental stress. This is the well-described fight or flight response, with increase in heart rate and other hormones (cortisol and growth hormone).

Catecholamine excess is seen in the syndrome of pheochromocytoma, discussed below. Hypofunction of the adrenal medulla is seldom clinically significant, since catecholamines are made in other sites of the body (e.g., sympathetic nervous chain).

CATECHOLAMINE EXCESS: PHEOCHROMOCYTOMA

Pheochromocytoma is a neuroendocrine tumor that produces excess catecholamines. It is usually a benign tumor, but can be malignant in rare cases. Most "pheos" occur within the adrenal medulla itself. It is an uncommon cause of hypertension, and for this reason it is sometimes a missed diagnosis. Although we all have occasional bursts of catecholamine excess when we are upset or are under stress, those with pheochromocytoma have it most of the time. During these severe episodes ("paroxysms") of excess, patients have numerous symptoms, such as diaphoresis, headache, tachycardia, pallor, and severe hypertension. These symptoms can be so severe that the patient dies of a stroke or myocardial infarction.

Pheochromocytoma may be diagnosed by several methods. The most common method is to measure catecholamines or their metabolites (metanephrines and vanillylmandelic acid (VMA)) in urine collected for a 24-hour period. "Spot" urine collections or serum measurements are less useful. After the presence of pheochromocytoma has been confirmed biochemically, localization studies (MRI or CT) should be done.

The treatment for most tumors is surgical excision. The patient must first be prepared with α-blocking agents (phenoxybenzamine), which help control the blood pressure. After adequate α-blockade has occurred, the heart rate may be slowed with β-blockers (propranolol).

GLUCOSE METABOLISM

REVIEW

In the last lecture we learned about the adrenal glands, which are also called the fight-or-flight glands. These glands secrete hormones that are necessary during physical stress and illness.

The two adrenal glands lie in the retroperitoneal cavity above the kidneys. The adrenal is divided into the outer adrenal cortex and the inner medulla. The adrenal cortex contains three layers that make steroid hormones. The steroids made by the adrenals include glucocorticoids, sex steroids, and mineralocorticoids. Sex steroid secretion is minimal when compared to those derived from the gonads.

Glucocorticoids are essential to life. They are called this because they increase glucose concentrations by increasing gluconeogenesis. The trophic hormone for glucocorticoid synthesis is the pituitary hormone ACTH—ACTH stimulation results in increased glucocorticoid synthesis, and decreased ACTH results in deficiency. The primary glucocorticoid of interest is cortisol (hydrocortisone).

Cushing's syndrome is a condition of cortisol excess. It may be caused by ACTH hypersecretion or be ACTH independent in nature. The most common cause of Cushing's syndrome is called Cushing's disease, a condition resulting from a pituitary tumor that secretes too much ACTH. Cushing's syndrome may also be caused by non-adrenal tumors that secrete ACTH. This is called ectopic ACTH syndrome. ACTH-independent causes of Cushing's syndrome include adrenal tumors and endogenous steroid ingestion. Clinical features of Cushing's syndrome include muscle weakness, excessive bruising, pigmented striae, central obesity, and a "moon face."

Adrenal insufficiency is the opposite of Cushing's syndrome and may be caused by a variety of conditions. Primary adrenal insufficiency is also called Addison's disease and usually results from autoimmune distraction of the adrenal gland. Secondary adrenal insufficiency may be caused by hypopituitarism. Patients who have been receiving exogenous glucocorticoids may develop adrenal insufficiency after the drugs are withdrawn too quickly.

Patients with Addison's disease have elevated ACTH levels, since this is a primary organ deficiency syndrome. This increased ACTH often results in a hyperpigmented appearance, because of the similarity of ACTH to melanocyte-stimulating hormone (MSH), important in lower animals. Other symptoms of adrenal insufficiency include anorexia, weakness, hypotension, and hyperkalemia. Adrenal insufficiency is easily treated with oral glucocorticoids.

The congenital adrenal hyperplasias (CAH) are a group of inherited disorders of steroid biosynthesis. These disorders may result in problems due to: (a) inadequate production of necessary steroids (e.g., cortisol); or (b) accumulation of steroid precursors with undesirable properties (e.g., androgens). The most common form is 21-hydroxylase deficiency, which may lead to masculinization of females and early virilization of males.

Mineralocorticoids are also made by the adrenal cortex. Aldosterone is the primary mineralocorticoid of interest and its synthesis is regulated by the reninangiotensin system, not the pituitary gland. Patients with primary adrenal insufficiency have mineralocorticoid deficiency and require replacement therapy. Hypopituitarism therefore does not result in significant mineralocorticoid deficiency, and patients with secondary adrenal insufficiency do not require mineralocorticoid replacement.

Aldosterone excess results in hyperaldosteronism. This in turn results in hypokalemia due to increased potassium excretion by the kidneys. Severe hypertension may also result. The most common cause of hyperaldosteronism is an adrenal tumor (benign or malignant). Treatment is surgical excision of the tumor. Most other cases of hyperaldosteronism are caused by bilateral hyperplasia, and these patients are best managed medically.

Renovascular hypertension is a relatively common cause of hypertension. This is caused by stenosis (blockage) of the renal artery, which fools the kidney into thinking that decreased blood flow is present. The kidney therefore tells the liver to produce more angiotensin II, resulting in a form of secondary hyperaldosteronism. This may be treated by correction of the stenotic lesion.

Finally, the adrenal medulla is important in synthesis of catecholamines. Catecholamines are also synthesized in other neural tissue. A disorder of clinical interest in the adrenal medulla is pheochromocytoma. Pheochromocytomas produce excess catecholamines and this may result in severe hypertension, stroke, and even death. These tumors are typically benign and usually unilateral, although bilateral tumors may occur. They are best treated by surgical excision.

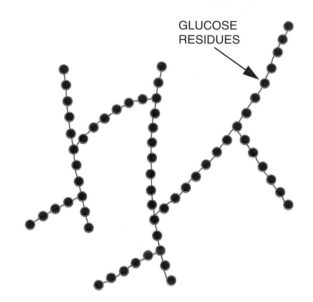

GLUCOSE RESIDUES

GLUCOSE METABOLISM

All living organisms require energy to survive. We obtain energy by ingesting fuels such as carbohydrates, protein, and lipids. This is called the anabolic (building) phase of energy metabolism. The body may also synthesize carbohydrates and lipids as needed. In the well-fed state, excess glucose is converted to glycogen, a compound made of multiple glucose molecules linked together. After the glycogen stores are filled, excess glucose is used for fatty acid synthesis. **Glucose is sort of like the "team manager" for our football team; it provides the energy (e.g., Gatorade) necessary for functions of the rest of the body.**

Problems result when disequilibrium between these two phases occurs. The risk of an inadequate anabolic phase (eating too little) is starvation and death, while excess anabolism (eating too much) results in energy excess and obesity. Obesity can only occur when energy expended is less than energy taken in. Overweight persons who declare they "eat hardly anything" would be violating fundamental laws of physics that state: (a) matter can neither be created nor destroyed; and (b) energy is proportional to mass. It is true, though, that many overweight persons have a low basal metabolic rate and do not expend much energy, making it difficult for them to lose weight.

The catabolic or breakdown state is necessary to maintain energy levels 4–6 hours after eating. The body's immediate energy needs can be met by glycogen breakdown to glucose. Glycogen stores, however, only last about 12 hours after fasting and cannot meet long-term energy needs. After that, fatty acid oxidation is required.

In this lecture, we will discuss the common disorders of glucose metabolism, such as diabetes mellitus.

INSULIN AND GLUCAGON

Understanding insulin is important in the study of glucose metabolism. Insulin is a protein hormone produced in the β (beta) cells of the pancreas. **Insulin starts out as the precursor molecule preproinsulin,** which is then cleaved to proinsulin in the cell. Proinsulin is next broken up into insulin and C-peptide

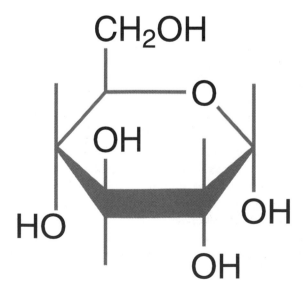

(connecting peptide); the latter appears to have no biological activity, although some have postulated that it may be of some biological significance.

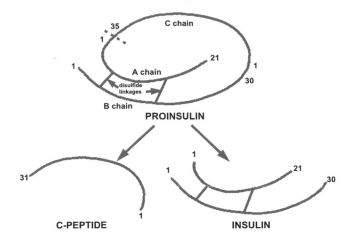

Insulin is an anabolic hormone that promotes energy storage. It promotes glycogen and fatty acid synthesis, glycolysis, and triglyceride storage, and inhibits glycogenolysis, hepatic ketogenesis, and gluconeogenesis. Insulin increases glucose transport across cell membranes by means of glucose transporters (GLUTs). Many different GLUTs have been identified; for example, GLUT-4 is found in muscle. Insulin levels rise in response to a sugar load, and decrease when levels return to normal. A basal amount of insulin is always necessary for maintenance of glucose homeostasis.

Glucagon is made in the α (alpha) cells of the pancreas, and is sort of an antagonist to insulin. Its function is catabolic (breaks down molecules to provide energy for cells), in contrast to insulin, which is anabolic in nature (builds molecules). Secretion is inhibited by high glucose and fatty acid levels, and stimulated by hypoglycemia. It is important in recovery from hypoglycemia, and some diabetics develop a loss of glucagon response to hypoglycemia. These patients keep injectable glucagon on hand for use in cases of severe hypoglycemia. The pancreatic hormone somatostatin (also made in the hypothalamus) inhibits secretion of both glucagon and insulin.

DIABETES MELLITUS

Diabetes mellitus (DM) is a disorder of glucose metabolism whose name is derived from the Greek words diabetes ('siphon') and mellitus ('sweet'), and was first described in an Egyptian papyrus dated 1500 B.C.

Ancient civilizations noted that ants were attracted to the high-glucose urine of diabetics. They also made a distinction between two types of diabetes. The first form occurred in children and young adults who were thin. These individuals essentially "wasted away" and died within a few years. This type of diabetes results from absence or deficiency of insulin and is called type 1 diabetes. Another, more indolent, form was described in older, overweight individuals. This is called type 2 diabetes and is caused by impaired insulin action (insulin resistance).

Diabetes is an extremely common disorder, affecting approximately 5% of the U.S. population. In the United States, type 2 is much more common, accounting for 90% of those with diabetes. The prevalence of type 2 has increased as obesity and sedentary lifestyles have become more common. The remaining 10% of diabetics have type 1 diabetes. This type is more common in northern European nations such as Sweden and Finland. Diabetes is an enormous economic problem—the estimated cost of diabetes and its complications is one out of every seven health care dollars.

Patients with diabetes cannot use glucose effectively, resulting in hyperglycemia. A large load of glucose is filtered through to the kidney, where water is carried with it. This results in the typical symptom of excessive urination (polyuria). Since the body loses too much water, excessive thirst (polydipsia) occurs. Finally, since the body cannot use glucose properly, it thinks it is in a starved state, and excessive eating (polyphagia) occurs. The body also breaks down fats and proteins in an effort to compensate for decreased energy utilization. In essence, then, the body is starved for fuel despite having too much of it! These three symptoms are called the "classic symptoms" of diabetes or "polys." Not all patients with diabetes have symptoms, however; many persons with type 2 are asymptomatic for years before diabetes is discovered on a routine screening test. There are three ways to diagnose diabetes: (1) two fasting serum glucose levels ≥126 mg/dL (7.0 mmol/L); (2) serum glucose level ≥200 mg/dL (11.1 mmol/L) 2 hours after a 75 gram glucose load; (3) classic symptoms of diabetes with serum glucose ≥200 mg/dL.

Impaired glucose tolerance is a term used to describe those whose glucose levels are not entirely normal but who do not meet the criteria above. They are in a gray area between normal and diabetic and were once called "borderline diabetics" (an outdated term).

Such a term implies that the condition is not important or not serious, and it is certainly a condition that warrants monitoring.

TYPE 1 DIABETES

This type is also called insulin-dependent diabetes mellitus, and results from the near total deficiency of insulin. We used to call it "juvenile diabetes," but this term is not appropriate today because, although it is more common in children and young adults, it may occur in older adults. As we will discuss later, type 2 diabetes may also occur in younger individuals. Type 1 is typically an autoimmune disease, resulting in destruction of pancreatic islet cells by anti-islet cell antibodies (ILA). Deficiency of insulin results in hyperglycemia, ketoacidosis, and death if untreated.

TYPE I (INSULIN-DEPENDENT) DIABETES

PATHOGENESIS: DESTRUCTION OF PANCREAS
IMMUNOLOGIC: MOST COMMON CAUSE (ANTI-ISLET CELL ANTIBODIES)

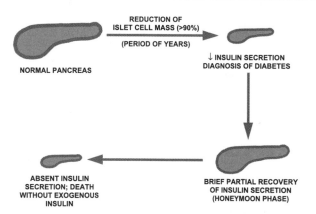

The typical patient with type 1 DM is a child or young adult with a several week period of weight loss, polyuria, polydipsia, and polyphagia. If this goes on too long without medical intervention, ketoacidosis will result. Prompt initiation of insulin therapy is necessary. As mentioned above, type 1 can occur in older adults, although type 2 is more common in this age group. A variant of type 1 occurring in adults is called LADA (latent autoimmune diabetes in adults). These are typically thin adults who respond poorly to oral therapy and require insulin.

After initial diagnosis, some insulin is still present in most new type 1 patients, and a brief state of remission often occurs in which symptoms and glucose levels normalize. This "honeymoon phase" is short-lived (typically several months) followed by absolute dependence on exogenous insulin.

Like all autoimmune diseases, type 1 diabetes appears to require both a genetic predisposition and an environmental trigger. Those with certain genetic (human leukocyte antigen or HLA) markers are predisposed to develop type 1 diabetes. But this alone is not enough—the environmental insult must also occur. For example, if one identical twin develops type 1 diabetes, the chance of the remaining twin developing it is only about 60%. If the second twin develops it, it may be much later in life than the first twin. This is in contrast to type 2 diabetes, where virtually 100% of twins either both develop the disorder, or neither develops it.

TYPE 2 DIABETES

This is the more common form of diabetes (90% of patients in the United States) and is often called non-insulin dependent diabetes or adult-onset diabetes. The latter term may be misleading, since type 2 can also occur in children, adolescents, or young adults. Indeed, the incidence of type 2 in these younger persons is increasing, as our society becomes more sedentary and overweight. A special variant of type 2 called MODY (maturity-onset diabetes of the young) may occur in young people. This is distinguished from typical type 2 diabetes in that MODY is usually inherited in autosomal dominant fashion and the typical patient has several first-degree relatives with ketosis-resistant diabetes that developed at a young age.

Unlike type 1, which is a state of insulin deficiency, type 2 is a state of hormone resistance in which insulin receptors lose their sensitivity to insulin. Insulin secretion initially is normal; in fact, insulin levels are often elevated early in the disorder, leading to hyperinsulinism. It is like having a big car with an 8-cylinder engine, and 6 of the spark plugs gone. The engine works very hard and burns a lot of gas, but does not drive the car very fast. This is in contrast to type 1, which is like a car with no gas. The end result is similar (the car does not go), but the pathophysiology is different. Many patients with type 2 are asymptomatic at the time of diagnosis and are diagnosed by routine screening.

TYPE 2 (NON-INSULIN DEPENDENT) DIABETES

PATHOGENESIS: INEFFECTIVE USE OF ENDOGENOUS INSULIN
EVENTUAL DECREASE OF BETA CELL MASS OVER YEARS

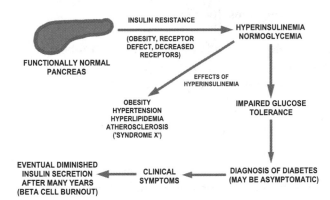

Most patients are overweight, which accounts for the insulin resistance. Populations that are traditionally lean (e.g., Asians) are more likely to develop the disease if they move to the United States and consume a typical high-calorie Western diet. About 15% of patients, however, are of normal body weight. Type 2 DM is an extremely heterogeneous disorder, with patients of all body shapes and sizes.

The evolutionary theory of natural selection postulates that deleterious genes are removed from the population because these persons die sooner and are less likely to reproduce. If this is true, then why is type 2 diabetes so common? We might theorize that at some point in time the tendency for type 2 might actually be advantageous. For most of our years of civilization, food was not always plentiful—life was hard and physically exhausting. Only the very wealthy had the luxuries of excess food and avoidance of physical labor. We know that many patients with type 2 diabetes are obese and gain weight easily with little food intake. These people might actually have an advantage in a society where food is scarce. Food, however, is abundant in most developed countries today, and this has made the tendency for type 2 disadvantageous. Physical activity has also diminished from our early years of civilization, contributing to obesity.

Many patients with type 2 diabetes are puzzled as to why their fasting glucose is often high in the morning. After all, they did not eat anything all night, so how could the morning glucose be high? This is explained by realizing that a cardinal derangement in type 2 diabetes is the presence of increased hepatic gluconeogenesis. Increased growth hormone secretion at night (the dawn phenomenon) also increases insulin resistance and contributes to fasting hyperglycemia. This is why many patients with type 2 benefit from an evening injection of insulin.

The tendency for type 2 DM appears to be inherited, but is not localized to specific chromosomal areas as is type 1 DM. The second, environmental trigger is not necessary (since type 2 is not an autoimmune disease). The person does, however, have some control over his or her destiny. Normalization of body weight early in life leads to less risk for diabetes. Genetic penetrance is quite high. If one identical twin has type 2 DM, the chance that the other will have it approaches 100%, assuming both have similar body sizes and health. In contrast, with type 1 DM, the likelihood of a second twin being affected is only about 60%.

HYPERINSULINEMIA AND SYNDROME X

The high insulin levels in our "inefficient engine" appear to do more than just result in hyperglycemia (if that wasn't enough!). Hyperinsulinemia appears to cause a vicious cycle of metabolic problems, including atherosclerotic disease, diabetes mellitus, hypertension, and hyperlipidemia (mainly hypertriglyceridemia).

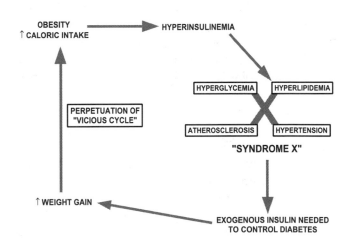

These problems may not present at the same time (e.g., a patient may experience hypertension and hypertriglyceridemia years before developing diabetes mellitus). Newer therapies for type 2 diabetes are directed at correcting the underlying problem of insulin resistance.

SECONDARY DIABETES

Secondary diabetes is diabetes caused by another condition. A common secondary form is caused by repeated episodes of pancreatitis (inflammation of the pancreas), which results in reduced β cell mass. Those who have undergone pancreatectomy obviously develop insulin deficiency and insulin-dependent diabetes. Infiltrative diseases may cause pancreatic destruction and diabetes. The most common cause is hemochromatosis, which results in excessive iron accumulation in visceral organs and pancreatic destruction. This is also called "bronze diabetes" because of the dark skin pigmentation due to iron accumulation. Drugs such as high-dose corticosteroids (e.g., prednisone) commonly cause hyperglycemia and diabetes.

GESTATIONAL DIABETES AND DIABETES IN PREGNANCY

Gestational diabetes (GDM) is yet another subset of diabetes. By definition, it develops during pregnancy, as opposed to type 1 or 2, which exist beforehand. The term usually refers to a state of reversible glucose intolerance that begins late in the second trimester of pregnancy. As the growing fetoplacental unit increases in size, substances such as human placental growth hormone and placental lactogen are secreted in large amounts, and increase insulin resistance. In susceptible individuals, gestational diabetes results. Risk factors include obesity, family history of type 2 diabetes, and advanced maternal age.

All pregnant women (except, of course, those who already have diabetes) should have a gestational diabetes screen at 24–26 weeks gestation. This is performed by giving a small glucose load (50 grams) and measuring serum glucose one hour afterwards. If the screen is positive, a formal glucose tolerance test (3 hours with a 100 gram glucose load) is then done. "Pure" gestational diabetes usually resolves after delivery. These persons do have a strong likelihood (about 50%) of developing type 2 diabetes later in life.

Good control of diabetes during pregnancy is essential (whether it is preexisting or gestational). Fetuses of mothers with preexisting diabetes may develop organ malformations if control in the first trimester is poor. This problem does not occur in those with gestational diabetes because the organs are already formed by the time the glucose intolerance occurs (after 26 weeks). Fetuses of mothers with both types of diabetes may develop macrosomia (a term meaning large babies). This may result in delivery problems due to their large size.

It is strongly recommended that patients with preexisting diabetes have excellent control before considering pregnancy. Adequate contraceptive measures are necessary in those without optimal control.

MONITORING DIABETES

Diabetes management is more advanced today than ever before. Much of the improvement of care is due to the invention of small, portable glucose meters. These are small, battery-powered devices that allow the user to check his or her blood glucose. This is done by applying a small drop of capillary blood (from pricking the fingertip) to a disposable strip then inserting into the meter. This gives the user a way to monitor his or her readings and adjust treatment as necessary. Some meters contain a computer chip that allow downloading of the readings into a computer for detailed analysis.

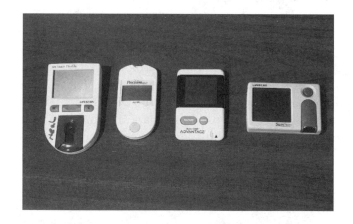

In the past, persons with diabetes monitored urine glucose. The first urine tests required boiling urine mixed with copper sulfate solution, which turned from blue to orange if glucose was present. Later, urine test strips became available. Urine glucose testing is not recommended today because of its inaccuracy, as the renal threshold for glucose varies among individuals. It may be used in patients who are unwilling to do self-monitoring of blood glucose (SMBG).

Treatment goals depend on the individual. It would be ideal to keep all diabetics within the normal range all the time, but this is not possible in most people.

One reason is that many treatments for diabetes (such as insulin) can cause hypoglycemia (low blood glucose). The tighter the control, the more likely such reactions are. While a young, healthy adult might tolerate hypoglycemia well, an older individual might fall down and break his leg, for instance.

A good rule of thumb is that the best degree of control without unacceptable hypoglycemia should be attained. Some will decide that they desire good diabetes control. Others, unfortunately, may not care much about their diabetes control and only wish to stay out of the hospital. Those with poor control are much more likely to develop complications than those with better control. It is like going to the appliance store to buy a washer and dryer. You can purchase the cheap version, which may work well for a few years, but then break down. Or, you can buy the mid-priced version, which will last for perhaps ten years. The top-of-the line model is the most expensive, but may last for a lifetime without breaking down. Diabetes control is the same way. Some of it boils down to luck. The cheap washer might last 25 years, but it probably won't. In the same line of thought, there are some patients with long histories of poorly controlled diabetes who have relatively few or no complications at all. Overall, the odds favor the person with well-controlled diabetes.

As mentioned, the glucose readings are the most important data for individuals with diabetes. On the other hand, one can only check so many times per day. It is possible that the person is high or low during times that were not checked. Therefore, it is useful to have a secondary, backup test used to correlate with the other tests. Fortunately, such a test exists and is called glycated hemoglobin (HbA_{1C}). This test measures the amount of hemoglobin (the protein that carries oxygen through the blood) that glucose attaches to, and is reported as a percentage of the total hemoglobin. It is a useful index of long-term diabetic control and accurately reflects blood glucose values for the last six weeks. It is good news if the patient's HbA_{1C} level correlates with the average of his or her blood glucose readings. If the HbA_{1C} is much higher than the glucose readings indicate, the patient may be having hyperglycemia at times not checked. If it is much lower than the glucose meter readings, he or she may be having frequent hypoglycemia. Or, the meter may not be working properly, or the patient may be lying about his or her readings (this is common!). Rarely, a patient may have abnormal hemoglobin molecules that do not allow an accurate reading (e.g., sickle cell

anemia, thalassemia). At this time, glycated hemoglobin is only recommended for use in established patients with diabetes, and not the diagnosis of diabetes itself.

How do we know that good diabetes control matters? Well, for years, we didn't...we just hoped that we were doing the right thing! Finally, in 1993, a study called the Diabetes Control and Complications Trial (DCCT) was completed. This study took many years to complete and studied 1500 patients with type 1 diabetes. Patients were randomized to receive either standard therapy (one or two injections per day—the mid-range model) or intensive therapy (multiple daily injections or insulin infusion pump—the deluxe model). It was shown that intensively treated patients had a lower incidence of many complications. The United Kingdom Prospective Diabetes Study (UKPDS) recently demonstrated similar findings in type 2 diabetics.

COMPLICATIONS OF DIABETES

Before effective treatments for diabetes were available, most patients died before they could develop complications. Even after insulin was discovered in 1921, it was many years before common complications were discovered. The initial exuberance over effective treatment of diabetes was later tempered by the recognition that complications developed in patients with poor control. These complications were more frequent in the early years of insulin therapy because blood glucose monitoring was not available.

Patients with diabetes are more prone to certain medical problems than normal people. These can be divided into two broad categories: microvascular (small vessel) and macrovascular (large vessel) disease. Microvascular diseases include diabetic retinopathy (eye disease), nephropathy (kidney disease), and neuropathy (nerve disease). Macrovascular disease includes coronary artery disease (angina pectoris and myocardial infarction), cerebrovascular disease (stroke), and peripheral vascular disease.

What causes the complications of diabetes? Although extremely high glucose levels may cause ketoacidosis and even death in severe circumstances, glucose itself does not appear to be the cause of chronic complications. The pathogenesis of diabetic complications remains poorly understood. Evidence indicates that many diabetic complications may be caused by advanced glycation end products (AGEs). Long-term hyperglycemia causes glycation of many proteins. These products themselves may cause protein damage dysfunction, or may cause production of deleterious products, such as tumor necrosis factor and interleukins.

DIABETIC NEUROPATHY

Neuropathy is a common complication of diabetes that can result in significant morbidity. It is divided into peripheral nerve (somatic) neuropathies, and autonomic (central nervous system) neuropathies. The most common form of neuropathy is a distal sensory neuropathy that results in distal numbness ("stocking" distribution). Pain may also occur with this type of neuropathy, and it may be resistant to treatment. A less common form of neuropathy is a proximal motor and sensory neuropathy (amyotrophy). A common form of autonomic neuropathy is hypoglycemia unawareness, in which the patient is unaware that his or her glucose is low. This may have devastating consequences, as the person may suffer a seizure, wreck a motor vehicle, or even die without intervention by another person. Sometimes autonomic neuropathies keep the patient's heart rate from increasing in response to exercise (fixed heart rate). Diabetic gastroparesis is another form of diabetic autonomic neuropathy that causes delayed gastric emptying. Because stomach contents are not readily emptied, nausea, vomiting, and early satiety (feeling full before the entire meal is eaten) may occur. Since food is absorbed erratically, poor diabetes control often develops. Medications are available that can help this problem.

The best treatment of diabetic neuropathy is improvement of glycemic control. Tricyclic antidepressants such as amitriptyline and anticonvulsants such as gabapentin and carbamazepine may be useful. Narcotic analgesics should be avoided, as they are not very effective and can be addicting.

THE DIABETIC FOOT

Patients with diabetes and peripheral vascular disease are much more likely to develop foot problems. A small abrasion or penetrating wound, while only a nuisance to normal persons, can be devastating to diabetics with these complications. An infected foot ulcer, for instance, can lead to weeks of hospitalization for antibiotic therapy or even amputation.

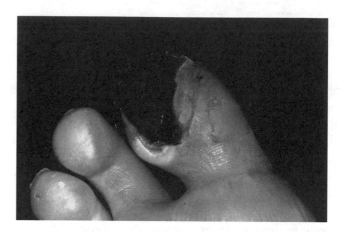

The health care provider should always look at the patient's feet during the examination. This often uncovers problems such as calluses or small ulcerations that were not previously known to the patient. Appropriate measures (e.g., antibiotics, referral to a podiatrist or pedorthist) are then possible before the problems become severe.

DIABETIC RETINOPATHY

Probably the most feared complication of diabetes is blindness. Millions of patients go blind each year as a result of this disease. With optimal control, however, the incidence of retinopathy decreases, and effective treatment is available.

There are two basic types of retinopathy: nonproliferative and proliferative. Nonproliferative or "background" retinopathy is seen in many patients after many years with diabetes. It does not cause vision loss, and if it does not progress, is of minimal significance in the peripheral visual field. It may cause problems in the central visual field (fovea) if macular edema (swelling in the foveal area) occurs.

Proliferative retinopathy is much more ominous. This leads to neovascularization (new blood vessel growth) and possible vitreous hemorrhage (bleeding into the eye) and retinal detachment. This may lead to vision loss and blindness. Fortunately, this can sometimes be prevented by laser photocoagulation (destroying new blood vessels in the peripheral field). This does not affect central vision. Peripheral and night vision may be slightly diminished by laser treatments.

All patients with diabetes must see a qualified optometrist or ophthalmologist on a regular basis to detect any new problems.

DIABETIC NEPHROPATHY

Diabetic nephropathy is another small vessel or microvascular disease, like retinopathy. Patients with diabetes for many years may begin to suffer early kidney damage. The first stage is manifested by hyperfiltration (increased filtration through the kidney). This is measured by performing a 24-hour urine collection for creatinine and measuring the creatinine clearance, which is a rough estimate of glomerular filtration rate (GFR). A normal value is between 70 and 120 ml/min. A patient with stage I nephropathy might have a creatinine clearance of, say, 180 ml/min. The initial response to your patient might be, "Fantastic! Your kidney function is 150% of normal! You have kidney function to spare!" This is, however, not fantastic at all; it is a harbinger of possible worsening of kidney disease. The kidney may also leak small amounts of protein, or microalbumin, at this point. Fortunately, the nephropathy is potentially reversible at this time with certain measures. A certain type of blood pressure medication, angiotensin converting-enzyme inhibitors (ACEI), help reverse nephropathy at this stage, even if the blood pressure is normal. As nephropathy progresses, microalbuminuria (small amounts of protein, <500 mg per day) persists. In the next stage, protein persists at over 500 mg per day (overt proteinuria), GFR decreases (meaning decreased kidney function), and hypertension occurs. At this stage, the kidney damage is clearly irreversible, and all patients will progress to complete kidney failure in time. Even at this late stage, however, the progression to complete failure can be slowed by good blood pressure and glucose control, and restriction of protein in the diet.

Those with end-stage nephropathy have complete kidney failure and will die without treatment. Available treatments include renal replacement therapy (dialysis) or kidney transplantation. Billions of dollars are spent yearly on dialysis treatments for diabetic patients, making this the most expensive diabetic complication to treat. One type of dialysis is called hemodialysis, in which the patient is connected to a dialysis machine by an arteriovenous fistula in the arm for several hours three times weekly. Another type is called CAPD (continuous ambulatory peritoneal dialysis). This works by using the peritoneal membrane of the abdomen as a filter. A catheter is placed permanently in the abdomen, and large amounts of peritoneal dialysis fluid are infused into this space. This process is much slower than hemodialysis because it works by passive diffusion. The large peritoneal dialysis bags are also quite cumbersome, but this procedure has the advantage of performing it at home. Some patients prefer this to hemodialysis. One problem with CAPD is that the dialysate (fluid) bags contain large amounts of glucose, which may interfere with diabetes control. Sometimes, insulin is placed in the CAPD bags, which may help control.

Life expectancy in diabetic dialysis patients is extremely poor, with the average survival after beginning therapy only 2 years. It appears that diabetics on dialysis have such severe vascular disease elsewhere that life expectancy is dismal. Good control of glucose and hypertension may help prolong survival.

Renal transplants are preferred in patients who are good candidates. Poor candidates include those who have severe cardiovascular disease and are morbidly obese (they might not tolerate surgery very well). The best transplants occur with a kidney from a related donor (e.g., a sibling). Living donors in good health may safely donate one kidney, as the remaining kidney is sufficient for them. Cadaveric (from a deceased donor) transplants are generally less successful than those from relatives. Patients undergoing transplantation need powerful anti-rejection drugs the rest of their lives. Those with successful transplants no longer require dialysis.

DIABETIC KETOACIDOSIS

Diabetic ketoacidosis (DKA) may occur in type 1 diabetics who are without insulin for long periods of time. In the normal person, basal insulin levels allow balanced glucose homeostasis. With lack of insulin, the body thinks it is in a starved state since glucose cannot get into the cells (when in fact the concentration in the blood is quite high). As a result, the body starts breaking down fats and proteins, producing waste products such as ketones in an effort to gain energy from these sources. This propagates a vicious cycle—the body has plenty of glucose in the blood, but cannot use it!

The breakdown products of these alternate energy sources (e.g., ketones) eventually result in ketoacidosis. Medium-chain ketones have a fruity odor, and the breath of these patients often smells fruity. The very high glucose concentration in the blood acts as an osmotic diuretic and causes massive fluid losses from the body via the urine. These patients are therefore very dehydrated in addition to being acidotic. Death results if untreated.

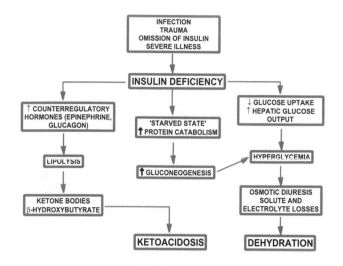

One of the most common reasons for ketoacidosis is infection (e.g., pneumonia, urinary tract infection). Another common cause is omission of insulin on sick days. Patients sometimes think that if they are sick and not eating, they should omit their insulin. Nothing is further from the truth! Even persons not eating need some insulin to maintain normal bodily functions. The ill person should instead follow sick day rules that involve taking the scheduled insulin plus supplemental soluble insulin every few hours if high.

Diabetic ketoacidosis (DKA) is treated with fluids and insulin. Large amounts of fluids (e.g., 5–10 liters) may be necessary to restore the lost fluids (i.e., with 0.9% normal saline). Older patients with diminished cardiac reserve may need special monitoring to prevent congestive heart failure and pulmonary edema.

Insulin is most commonly administered as an intravenous infusion for DKA, and is continued until the acidosis resolves. Subcutaneous insulin must be started at least an hour before the intravenous insulin is discontinued, due to the latter's short half-life (under 10 minutes).

HYPEROSMOLAR NONKETOTIC SYNDROME (HNKS)

The hyperosmolar nonketotic syndrome (HNKS) is another syndrome of acute metabolic decompensation in diabetics. Like DKA, these patients have severe hyperglycemia (often >1000 mg/dL) and dehydration; unlike DKA, ketoacidosis is absent. HNKS is commonly the presenting manifestation of diabetes in elderly patients and is typically associated with a concurrent illness (e.g., infection, myocardial infarction, stroke).

HNKS differs from DKA since patients with the former have sufficient insulin to prevent lipolysis and metabolic acidosis. However, there is enough relative insulin deficiency to cause hyperglycemia and protein/carbohydrate catabolism, leading to osmotic diuresis with fluid and electrolyte depletion.

The treatment of HNKS includes fluid and electrolyte repletion. Intravenous insulin is also necessary in most patients. Subcutaneous insulin is started after the acute metabolic decompensation resolves, and underlying conditions such as infection are treated.

THERAPY OF TYPE 1 DIABETES

Patients with type 1 diabetes had a dismal future before the discovery of insulin. All patients died, and life could be miserably prolonged a year or two by administering starvation diets that deprived the patient of glucose. It was discovered in 1889 that total pancreatectomy produced diabetes in dogs, and the concept of a glucose-lowering substance located in the pancreatic islets of Langerhans was postulated. After many years of fruitless investigation, insulin was discovered in 1921 at the University of Toronto by Fred Banting (a surgeon); Charles Best (a medical student); James Collip (a biochemist); and J.J.R. Macleod (a physiologist). Banting and Macleod received the Nobel Prize for their efforts. Their insulin was soluble or regular insulin (pure human insulin without any additives). When injected as a subcutaneous depot, its onset of action is 0.5 to 2 hours, with a peak in 3–4 hours and duration of 6–8 hours; it is therefore termed short-acting or rapid-acting insulin. While lifesaving to millions of diabetics, the short duration of action was inconvenient.

It was then discovered that the addition of certain impurities to regular insulin resulted in delayed absorption. This gave birth to the intermediate- and long-acting series of insulins. One retarding agent is zinc, used in the Lente series (Lente, Ultralente, Semilente). Another is the protein protamine, used in NPH (also called N) insulin. Ultralente is a very long-lasting human insulin, with a peak of about 12–16 hours. A new insulin preparation, insulin glargine, has recently become available. This insulin lasts for over 24 hours and may be useful as a basal insulin. Most patients with type 1 diabetes require a mixture of rapid-acting and intermediate- or long-acting insulin.

Insulin is a large peptide hormone that unfortunately is rapidly degraded in the gastrointestinal tract, making oral administration difficult. At this time it must be given subcutaneously (under the skin). Depending on the preparation, subcutaneous absorption may take place within minutes or within hours. Some preparations last almost an entire day. Intravenous insulin administration is impractical, as the short half-life of insulin in serum requires a continuous infusion for efficacy.

Insulin is also well absorbed through the peritoneal cavity and may be administered this way in certain patients (e.g., those on dialysis). Other methods of insulin administration (e.g., inhaled aerosol) are being studied experimentally.

In the last decade, scientists have sought more rapid-acting insulins. Regular (R) insulin sometimes lasts for 4–6 hours, producing unpredictable hypoglycemia in certain patients. By synthetically modifying human insulin, rapid insulin analogs were discovered. The first such insulin, lispro, takes action in only 15 minutes and peaks in 30 minutes to 1 hour. This insulin is advantageous since it may be taken right before a meal (versus 30 minutes for R insulin). Another synthetic insulin, aspart insulin, has similar properties.

For many decades, insulin was produced from beef and hog pancreases. Although these proteins differ slightly from human insulin, they work well in humans. Since they are foreign proteins, however, a small percentage of people developed allergic reactions to animal insulins. Another concern was that the supply of animal pancreases might someday be exhausted, leading to inadequate insulin supplies. For these reasons, almost all insulin available today is synthetic human insulin of recombinant DNA origin. It is made by inserting the gene for human insulin into bacteria or yeast, which then manufacture the insulin.

DIET THERAPY

Good nutrition is as important as medication for good control of diabetes. In those with type 2 diabetes, it is the preferred initial therapy (those with type 1 also need insulin). Unfortunately, many patients who are willing to take insulin or pills are unable or unwilling to follow a diet. The most feared professional in the diabetes clinic is often not the physician, but the mean dietitian, who asks patients to make dietary modifications. Fortunately, diet prescriptions (yes, food is like a drug to a person with diabetes) are more flexible today than ever before. In the past, they were very rigid and

required patients to weigh food. Now they center on total amounts of calories and food groups. The diet should be tailored to the patient—some may be unable to follow an excessively complex diet plan.

The simplest way of following a sensible diet is the food pyramid. Foods at the top of the pyramid should be eaten sparingly or not at all (high fat foods, desserts, alcoholic beverages). Those at the bottom (e.g., cereals) can be eaten in much larger portions. This is a relatively simple plan that most people can follow.

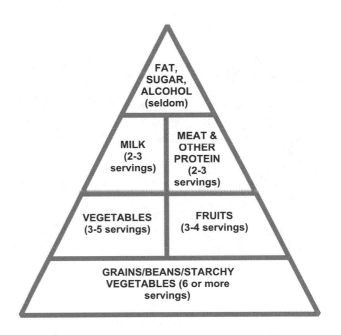

An exchange list diet is a method where foods are grouped into carbohydrate, meat/meat substitute, and fat groups. Exchange lists are a simple way of making food choices. Each person can eat a certain number from each exchange for each meal. For example, if another carbohydrate is desired, the person simply makes a substitution for the equivalent amount of another exchange.

Patients with type 2 diabetes are often overweight and the goal is a modest weight loss. Weight loss of one to two pounds per week is desired.

INSULIN PUMPS

Many patients with diabetes, including a recent Miss America, use insulin pumps. These devices supply insulin via continuous subcutaneous insulin infusion (CSII), a method by which short-acting insulin is continuously infused by the pump. Pumps are small, beeper-sized devices that contain insulin, and deliver it to the patient through a thin plastic tube inserted under the skin at the one end. An implantable pump has been studied experimentally. This is implanted inside the body, like a pacemaker, and is refilled periodically with insulin delivered through a subcutaneous infusion port. This is programmed with an external device much in the same way as an external pump, and the insulin is released into the peritoneal cavity (where it is absorbed almost as rapidly as intravenous insulin). These are not currently available for commercial use.

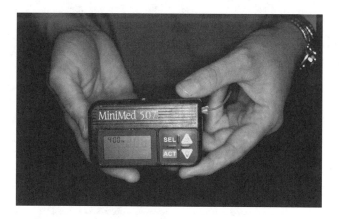

The patient programs the external pump to give a set amount of basal insulin, and gives additional insulin (boluses) before meals. The advantage of the pump is that very small amounts of insulin can be given accurately (in increments of 0.1 units). With conventional syringes, insulin can be given only in 1-unit increments.

There are misconceptions about pumps. A commonly held notion is that the pump gives insulin by itself without intervention by the wearer. The basal rate function does give insulin continuously, but the user has to set it. And meal boluses are not given without user instruction. The pump has no way of knowing what the wearer's glucose is, and so this must be checked in the same way as always (with a glucose meter). Pump therapy is actually much more complicated and expensive than conventional injections. In return, however, it allows more flexibility.

It is like comparing a Chevrolet sedan to an Indianapolis 500 race car. Conventional insulin injections are like the Chevy: almost anybody can drive it acceptably under typical conditions. But this vehicle lacks the flexibility to deal with unusual situations.

The Indy race car, on the other hand, can go over 200 miles per hour and is a much more sophisticated machine. Without adequate training, however, the average person driving it is likely to have a wreck. The same is true with a pump—those poorly suited for a pump are likely to have more problems than they did using injections.

Pumps are generally only for patients with type 1 diabetes, although some type 2s with low insulin requirements may benefit. Current pumps are unable to deliver the large amounts of insulin necessary for very insulin resistant individuals. Also, patients with type 2 diabetes are much less prone to hypoglycemia and therefore do not often require the benefits of the pump.

TEAM APPROACH TO DIABETES

Good diabetes treatment usually requires more than what the physician can provide. Unlike many other medical disorders, the patient has to do most of the work; it is not as simple as taking a pill. This requires that patients be well educated about their illness. The diabetes team may consist of the following: Physician; diabetes educator; nurse practitioner; registered dietitian; podiatrist; ophthalmologist/optometrist; vascular surgeon; nephrologist; social worker; and mental health/ counseling services.

A Certified Diabetes Educator (CDE) should be the primary educational resource in teaching patients about diabetes care. These are health care professionals (physicians, registered nurses, dietitians, or pharmacists) who have an interest, and have received advanced training, in the care and education of patients with diabetes. They must take a rigorous qualifying examination and be periodically recertified.

ORAL AGENTS FOR DIABETES

In addition to insulin, there are many oral agents. These are often called oral hypoglycemic agents or antihyperglycemic agents. The oral agents can be divided into several classes.

Sulfonylureas were first discovered in the 1940s during World War II when new antibiotics were being developed. Researchers found that several patients receiving the experimental antibiotics suffered hypoglycemia. Carbutamide was the first sulfonylurea used but had adverse clinical effects. The so-called first-generation agents were introduced in the late 1950s and included tolbutamide and chlorpropamide. Acetohexamide and tolazamide were introduced later. The second-generation sulfonylureas were then introduced; these include glyburide and glipizide. The newest second-generation agent is glimepiride.

Sulfonylureas act by sensitizing the pancreatic beta cells to glucose, and this results in increased insulin secretion. Intact beta cells are required, and so they are not useful in type 1 diabetics (who completely lack exogenous insulin).

Since sulfonylureas are insulin secretagogues, hypoglycemia may occur. Patients with prolonged hypoglycemia require admission to the hospital due to the relatively long duration of action of sulfonylureas. Chlorpropamide, specifically, has a very long half-life and should be used with caution.

Another class of drugs, the meglinitides, are derivatives of benzoic acid, and include repaglinide and natiglinide. Although structurally different than sulfonylureas, it acts in a similar fashion and may be thought of as a fast-acting sulfonylurea. It is generally taken before meals. Because it increases insulin secretion, it also may produce hypoglycemia. Meglinitides may be combined with other oral agents or insulin.

Biguanides are a class of drugs that increase insulin sensitivity and decrease hepatic glucose output. Metformin is a biguanide and a very useful drug for the treatment of type 2 diabetes. It may be used by itself or in combination with other oral agents or insulin. Metformin, because it does not increase insulin secretion, does not cause hypoglycemia. It may increase the effectiveness of other agents (such as insulin and sulfonylureas), and may potentiate the hypoglycemic effects of these drugs. Its most common adverse side effect is gastrointestinal: it occasionally causes mild diarrhea and increased flatulence. Only rarely, however, is this severe enough to necessitate discontinuation of the drug.

The most serious side effect of metformin therapy is lactic acidosis, which is fortunately quite rare (less than 1 per 30,000). Metformin increases the body's lactic acid production to a slight extent, and this is of no consequence in normal persons. In those with significant kidney or liver disease, though, this complication can occur rarely, and may result in death. This drug therefore should not be used in such patients. It is a very safe drug in normal patients without these problems.

A novel class of drugs is the thiazolidinedione (TZD or glitazone) class. These drugs act by increasing the body's sensitivity to insulin, thus attacking the fundamental problem in patients with type 2 diabetes. The two drugs currently available include pioglitazone and rosiglitazone. Troglitazone has been associated with hepatic disease in rare cases and was taken off the market in the United States in early 2000. This side effect has so far not been observed with the other drugs. Because of the experience with troglitazone, however, routine serum liver enzyme studies are recommended in patients taking the other TZD drugs.

The α-glucosidase inhibitors are the final class of oral agents. These drugs (acarbose and miglitol) inhibit α-glucosidase, an enzyme found in the brush border of the small intestine. These drugs inhibit the absorption of sucrose (but not lactose) and more complex sugars. This effectively leads to decreased absorption of these sugars after a meal. Glucose absorption is not affected. A frequent side effect of acarbose or miglitol therapy is increased flatulence, due to colonic bacterial digestion of the unabsorbed substances. They are useful in selected type 2 diabetics with elevated postprandial glucose levels.

CURING AND PREVENTING DIABETES

Diabetes is a tremendous medical and economic burden on the patient and society. Approximately one out of every seven health care dollars is spent on diabetes and its complications. It should consequently be no surprise that there are many efforts under way to cure or prevent this disease.

From a theoretical perspective, type 1 diabetes seems simplest to cure. All that is necessary is to replace insulin in a physiologic fashion. This is, of course, easier said than done—current therapies only provide an approximation of what a normal person's body does.

The closest thing to a cure for type 1 diabetes is restoration of the patient's beta cell mass by transplantation of the whole pancreas (pancreas transplantation) or of the islets themselves (islet cell transplantation). In whole pancreas transplantation, a cadaveric organ is used (a living donor is of course impossible, as that person needs his or her pancreas). Islet cell transplantation is more difficult; this involves purification of islets from a donor and infusing them into the portal vein. These functional islets set up shop in the liver and begin sensing glucose levels and secreting insulin, just as if they were in the pancreas. The advantage of these procedures is the achievement of normal or near-normal glycemic control with freedom from insulin, thus reducing the likelihood of long-term complications and improving the quality of life. Unfortunately, both the foreign pancreas and islet cells will be rejected by the recipient's immune system without potent immunosuppressive drugs. Researchers in Canada, however, have had initial success with islet cell transplantation using a steroid-free regimen. Because of the risks of these potent drugs, pancreas and islet cell transplants are usually reserved for patients who also require another organ (e.g., a kidney). Because immunosuppressive drugs would be required anyway, transplantation carries little additional risk. Nonetheless, several centers are now performing pancreas-only transplantation for those with severe diabetic complications. The five-year survival of a whole pancreas transplant is about 60%, while islet cell graft longevity is lower. In any case, patients with a functional graft have a significantly better quality of life than before. A better understanding of ways to overcome immune rejection will lead to improved survival of these grafts. Even if the immune problems can be solved, though, there are far too few donor pancreases or pancreatic islets to meet the needs of the millions with type 1 diabetes.

Another approach is to improve insulin pumps into truly "closed-loop" systems. Currently, the pumps require a great deal of intervention by the wearer (checking blood glucose, programming insulin boluses). It would be wonderful if an implantable insulin sensor were available that provided feedback to the pump with fewer necessary interventions. At this time, sensors that survive in the body for long periods of time are not available but are being studied experimentally.

Several clinical trials have also examined the prospects of preventing the development of type 1 diabetes. First-degree relatives of those with type 1 DM may enroll in these trials, and they are monitored for development of islet cell autoantibodies and/or hyperglycemia. Individuals who develop autoantibodies and hyperglycemia may receive an immunosuppressive drug, which appears to at least delay the onset of type 1 diabetes. Some patients also may receive oral insulin. Although not very effective as a treatment for diabetes, oral insulin may induce immune tolerance in some patients and delay the deleterious effects of the autoantibodies on the pancreas.

HYPOGLYCEMIA

"Hypoglycemia" is often a disorder poorly understood by physicians and other health care providers, as well as patients. Many patients casually note during the history that they or another family member has "low blood sugar," and needs to keep something around to eat at all times. In reality, hypoglycemia is an extraordinarily rare disorder that most providers are unlikely to encounter, except in the instance of insulin- or sulfonylurea-treated diabetics. It is a commonly touted cause of societal ills in the lay press, and many sources in print and on the Internet exist to propagate the notion of this disorder.

When most people think of hypoglycemia, they think of postprandial or reactive hypoglycemia. The normal response to an oral glucose load is secretion of an appropriate amount of insulin by the pancreas, resulting in euglycemia. In those with true reactive hypoglycemia, the insulin response is exaggerated, leading to postprandial hypoglycemia with resultant symptoms. True reactive hypoglycemia is quite rare, and often over-diagnosed, usually by misuse of the 100-gram glucose tolerance test. Even if reactive hypoglycemia does exist, it is not a life-threatening disorder, not a cause of constant fatigue and suffering, and may be managed with smaller, more frequent meals and avoidance of concentrated sweets.

Patients with abnormal gastric emptying (e.g., post-gastrectomy) have rapid "dumping" of food into the intestinal tract, which may result in hyperinsulinism. They may in fact have severe postprandial hypoglycemia. Treatment involves smaller, more frequent meals.

Another important note is that those persons with impaired glucose tolerance occasionally have delayed insulin release one or two hours after a meal, resulting in mild postprandial hypoglycemia. Treatment is weight loss and dietary management. It is common for a patient with type 2 diabetes to mention that he or she had "hypoglycemia" when younger.

A much more ominous form of hypoglycemia is fasting hypoglycemia, which occurs in the patient who has gone without food for several hours. Typically the patient feels worst in the morning and feels better after eating. This type of hypoglycemia is associated with either insulin hypersecretion or glucose underproduction.

An insulin-secreting islet cell tumor (insulinoma) is a rare cause of fasting hypoglycemia. These patients are prone to spontaneous attacks of weakness, hypoglycemic symptoms, and even syncope, seizures, and death if untreated. Treatment involves removal of the offending tumor. Other tumors can produce hypoglycemia by a yet-unidentified humoral factor.

Another important cause of hypoglycemia is factitious use of hypoglycemic agents (insulin or sulfonylureas). These persons usually have some type of psychiatric problem and derive some secondary gain from these attacks (e.g., sympathy from family, time off from work). Surreptitious insulin use can be distinguished from insulinoma by measuring C-peptide levels. Since endogenous insulin is produced by the cleavage of proinsulin to insulin and C-peptide, the plasma levels of both are elevated; with injection of exogenous insulin, only the insulin level is elevated. Sulfonylureas increase endogenous insulin secretion, so the C-peptide test is not useful in this instance. Urine or plasma drug tests for sulfonylureas may be valuable in these cases.

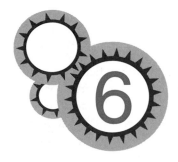

CALCIUM METABOLISM

REVIEW

Let's review what we learned in the last lecture. Insulin is an important hormone in glucose metabolism. It is made by pancreatic β cells and is cleaved from a precursor molecule called proinsulin. Glucagon is another hormone of somewhat lesser importance in glucose metabolism. Glucagon is made in the α cells and is an antagonist to insulin, and therefore important in recovering from hypoglycemia. Insulin is an anabolic hormone that promotes energy storage, while glucagon is a hormone that is catabolic (breaks down molecules).

Diabetes mellitus is a common disorder of glucose metabolism, and may be divided into type 1 and type 2. Type 1 is an autoimmune disease and results from the absence or deficiency of insulin and is more commonly seen in children and young adults, although older individuals can develop type 1. These patients require insulin in order to live. Type 2 diabetes is much more common and is primarily a disorder of insulin resistance in which the body uses insulin ineffectively. Most patients with type 2 are obese. Insulin may be required for adequate glucose control in patients with type 2 diabetes, although it is not necessary for life. Impaired glucose tolerance is a term used for patients whose blood glucose levels lie in the gray area between normal and high enough to meet the criteria for diabetes. Many of these patients develop diabetes in later life.

The insulin resistance and hyperinsulinemia of type 2 diabetes ("syndrome X") are very harmful to the body. These factors contribute to the increased incidence of hypertension, cardiovascular disease, obesity, and hyperlipidemia in patients with type 2 diabetes.

Gestational diabetes is diabetes that occurs during pregnancy. This term usually refers to patients who develop a reversible state of glucose intolerance during the late second to third trimester of gestation. Glucose tolerance usually returns to normal after delivery, although many of these persons develop type 2 diabetes later in life. Patients with pre-existing type 1 and type 2 diabetes also may become pregnant, and good glucose control in all pregnant individuals with diabetes is extremely important to prevent complications.

One of the cornerstones of diabetes management is the self blood-glucose monitor. Patients obtain a sample of capillary blood and place it on a small strip that gives them a glucose reading in seconds. Another important tool in diabetes management is the glycated hemoglobin (HbA$_{1c}$) level. This provides an index of glycemic control over the previous six weeks and is a useful adjunct to self-blood glucose monitoring. There is now substantial evidence that good diabetes control helps prevent complications as demonstrated by the DCCT and the UKPDS clinical trials.

Patients with diabetes are prone to develop many complications. These may be divided into the microvascular (small blood vessel) and macrovascular (large blood vessel) syndromes. Diabetic neuropathy is a type of microvascular complication in which nerve cells are damaged. The most common type of diabetic neuropathy results in numbness in both feet. This may result in patients developing ulcers because of lack of sensation. Other types of neuropathy are less common.

Diabetic retinopathy is another form of microvascular disease and is a substantial cause of blindness in society. Non-proliferative retinopathy is less serious and normally requires only routine surveillance. Proliferative retinopathy is more ominous and may lead to bleeding inside the eye, retinal detachment, and blindness. This may be treated by laser photocoagulation of the new blood vessels and surgery if necessary.

Diabetic nephropathy is yet another microvascular complication and is heralded by an increase in the glomerular filtration rate. Elevation of urine microalbumin is seen next, followed by a slow decline in glomerular filtration rate and fixed proteinuria. Diabetic nephropathy may be reversible if detected in the early stages. A minority of patients with diabetic nephropathy will develop end-stage renal disease and require renal replacement therapy (dialysis or renal transplantation). End-stage renal disease is the most expensive complication of diabetes to treat.

Diabetic ketoacidosis occurs in patients with type 1 diabetes who lack adequate insulin to meet metabolic needs. This is a vicious cycle in which the body thinks it is starved because it cannot use glucose, when in fact glucose in the serum is actually quite high. The elevated glucose leads to dehydration because of osmotic diuresis, and catabolic hormones such as glucagon and epinephrine worsen the problem leading to catabolism of fat and protein, and production of ketone bodies and ketoacids. This condition results in death if untreated. Treatment involves intravenous insulin and fluids. Hyperosmolar nonketotic syndrome is similar to ketoacidosis but is usually seen in older individuals without total insulin deficiency. These patients have elevated serum glucose levels but do not develop acidosis.

The only therapy for type 1 diabetes is insulin. At this time, insulin must be injected into the body, although experimental insulin delivery methods such as inhaled insulin are being studied. Most patients with type 1 diabetes take a combination of short-acting insulin and long- or intermediate-acting insulin. Insulin pumps are also used for patients with type 1 diabetes. An insulin pump is a small external device that delivers insulin continuously to the patient by means of a small plastic catheter. These devices are somewhat complicated and require a great deal of compliance for successful use. Nevertheless, studies show increased glucose control and fewer complications in motivated patients on pump therapy. Transplants of either a whole pancreas or pancreatic islet cells have been shown to be beneficial in select patients with difficult-to-control diabetes. A disadvantage of this type of therapy is the necessity of taking potent immunosuppressive drugs.

Treatment for type 2 diabetes may include diet therapy, oral agents, or insulin. Oral agents may be divided into four different categories. The first includes the insulin secretagogues, such as the sulfonylureas and meglinitides. These agents increase insulin secretion by the pancreas and therefore can potentially cause hypoglycemia. All other types of oral agents do not cause hypoglycemia. Metformin is a biguanide derivative that decreases hepatic glucose output and increases insulin sensitivity. A rare side effect of this medication is lactic acidosis that occurs rarely in patients with renal and/or hepatic insufficiency. The thiazolidinediones are novel drugs that increase insulin sensitivity. Finally, the alpha-glucosidase inhibitors decrease absorption of disaccharides and small polysaccharides by the small intestine, leading to decreased glucose levels after meals.

Hypoglycemia is a disorder that in fact is quite rare. It was believed in the past to be quite common, probably due to overuse of the glucose tolerance test. True reactive hypoglycemia is actually quite rare in the absence of structural gastrointestinal tract abnormalities. Insulinoma is a pathological cause of hypoglycemia—patients have spontaneous hypoglycemia and may develop seizures and even die if untreated. Another important cause of hypoglycemia is the factitious use of insulin and oral hypoglycemic agents, seen sometimes in patients with psychiatric disorders. Laboratory studies sometimes can help distinguish between endogenous and factitious causes of hypoglycemia.

TRANSPORT AND REGULATION OF CALCIUM

Although calcium lacks the glamour of the other hormones, it is important in many processes, including muscle contraction, synaptic transmission in the nervous system, platelet aggregation, coagulation, and secretion of hormones (as an intracellular second messenger). Unlike most of the hormones we have discussed, it is not under direct control by the pituitary gland or hypothalamus and is sort of like the "special team" squad on our football team.

Like iodothyronine hormones and sex steroids, the divalent cation calcium travels bound to serum proteins (such as albumin). About one-half is bound to proteins or other substances, while the remaining half circulates as free (sometimes called ionized) calcium. Like other hormones, it is the free, or unbound, moiety that is biologically active.

CALCIUM IN PLASMA

	mg/dL	mmol/L
TOTAL	8.4-10.1	2.2-2.5
IONIZED 46%	4.1-4.7	1.0-1.2
PROTEIN-BOUND 46%	4.1-4.7	1.0-1.2
COMPLEXED TO IONS 8%	0.7-0.8	0.18-0.2

Ionized calcium = active form

Total calcium is influenced by amount of serum proteins

Corrected Ca^{2+} = Measured Ca^{2+} + (0.8)(4 - serum albumin)

Calcium is not a classical hormone since it is not secreted from a gland; instead, it comes from several different sources. The largest supply of calcium is the skeleton, which houses over 99% of the body's calcium as a calcium phosphate salt. Dietary calcium also may be absorbed by the small intestine. The kidney plays an important role in reabsorbing calcium that is present in the blood and filtered through the urinary system.

The primary regulator of calcium metabolism is parathyroid hormone, secreted by the parathyroid glands. These small but mighty glands are pea-sized and usually located posterior to the thyroid gland. Most people have four parathyroids, but occasionally people have fewer or greater. An occasional individual may have a parathyroid located in another location, such as the mediastinum.

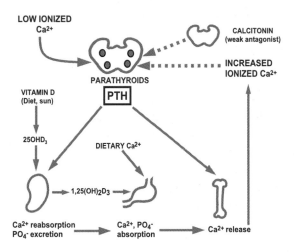

When serum calcium becomes low, this signals an increase in parathyroid hormone (PTH) levels. There are three actions of PTH that help restore serum calcium to normal.

1. Increased resorption of calcium from bone
2. Increased reabsorption of calcium from the kidney
3. Increased calcium absorption from the intestine

PTH has no direct effect on the intestine. It indirectly increases absorption due to its ability to increase the concentration of active vitamin D metabolites.

When calcium and PTH levels are normal, PTH actually enhances formation of bone. It is only with elevation of PTH levels that bone resorption occurs.

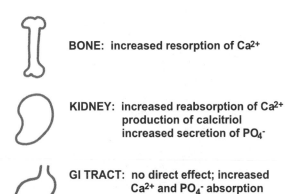

BONE: increased resorption of Ca^{2+}

KIDNEY: increased reabsorption of Ca^{2+} production of calcitriol increased secretion of PO_4^-

GI TRACT: no direct effect; increased Ca^{2+} and PO_4^- absorption via vitamin D

Vitamin D is also important in calcium metabolism. It is derived from cholesterol and is a sterol hormone formed from photogenesis in the skin and absorption from food. The photoconversion of sterol precursors to vitamin D was discovered in 1924, when scientists found that irradiation of an animal or its food prevented rickets in the animal. Even a small amount of sun exposure is enough to ensure adequate vitamin D stores (excessive sun exposure is not recommended!). Vitamin D itself has little activity but is converted to various activated metabolites. One of the major ones is calcidiol. The most important step in vitamin D metabolism is the conversion of calcidiol to calcitriol in the kidney. Calcitriol is the most active metabolite of vitamin D and its primary effect is increasing calcium and phosphorus absorption in the intestine. Vitamin D receptors are present in other organs but their role is less important. Hypocalcemia increases and hypercalcemia inhibits synthesis of calcitriol.

Calcitonin is a small protein secreted by the parafollicular (C) cells of the thyroid (as opposed to T4 and T3, which are made in the follicular cells). It is a weak antagonist of PTH and is secreted in response to hypercalcemia. Calcitonin is very important in salt-water animals (e.g., fish) that live in a high-calcium environment, but its importance is negligible in humans.

HYPERCALCEMIA

Mild hypercalcemia may present without symptoms. Moderate to severe hypercalcemia usually presents with symptoms of neuromuscular suppression. In general, symptoms include dehydration, weight loss, anorexia, pruritus, and polydipsia. Patients may also present with nausea, vomiting, fatigue, lethargy, confusion, and in severe cases, coma.

HYPERPARATHYROIDISM

The most common cause of hypercalcemia in the asymptomatic adult is primary hyperparathyroidism, with an incidence of 1 in 1000 patients. Most patients are asymptomatic and are detected only through routine screening. This condition results when one or more abnormally functioning glands secrete too much PTH, which causes increased reabsorption of calcium by the kidney, increased release of calcium by bone, and increased calcium absorption from the gut

(indirectly via vitamin D). Because increased PTH levels cause increased phosphate excretion (phosphaturia), serum phosphorus is decreased.

Most cases of primary hyperparathyroidism are due to a solitary parathyroid adenoma. The rest are usually due to hyperplasia of all four glands. Parathyroid carcinoma is a very rare and aggressive form of hyperparathyroidism.

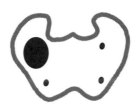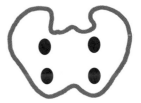

SOLITARY ADENOMA	HYPERPLASIA
REMAINING GLANDS	ALL FOUR GLANDS
SUPPRESSED	ENLARGED

At this time, there is no effective medical treatment for hyperparathyroidism. Estrogens may have minimal effect in postmenopausal women and may be tried. Anti-PTH analogs are being studied experimentally. The treatment of choice for primary hyperparathyroidism is therefore surgical excision of one or more abnormal parathyroid glands. In patients with a solitary adenoma, it is removed. In hyperplasia, the majority of all four glands is removed. Patients with asymptomatic disease and minimal calcium elevation often do not require surgery.

If surgery has been elected, several localization procedures may be useful prior to the procedure. At this time, the best test utilizes technetium-labeled sestamibi, a substance often used in nuclear cardiology. This procedure helps the surgeon localize the abnormal parathyroid gland(s) prior to surgery, which may decrease surgical time. Like a thyroid scan, it is not a diagnostic test; diagnosis still relies on serum biochemistry.

Patients with renal insufficiency may develop a different type of hyperparathyroidism. These patients often develop hypocalcemia because of decreased calcium reabsorption, chronic phosphate retention, and diminished production of calcitriol. This long-standing hypocalcemia results in elevated PTH levels that have no effect on the kidney, but still have effect on bone. Over time, these elevated PTH levels can cause bone resorption and bone pain. Treatment requires restriction of dietary phosphate, phosphate binding agents, and calcitriol to help increase the serum calcium. Since the hyperparathyroidism has been precipitated by another cause, it is called secondary hyperparathyroidism.

If this condition progresses too long, the parathyroid gland hypersecretion becomes autonomous, and persists even after calcium is brought into the normal range. This is called tertiary hyperparathyroidism and is difficult to manage. In this disorder, the only current therapy is removal of most of the parathyroid glands, since secretion is autonomous.

MALIGNANCY-ASSOCIATED HYPERCALCEMIA

Most patients with severe hypercalcemia have cancer, and the most common cause of malignancy-related hypercalcemia is humoral hypercalcemia of malignancy (HHM). The most common specific tumor-type is squamous cell lung carcinoma, although breast carcinoma, renal cell carcinoma, and bladder carcinoma may also be causes. We usually associate ectopic endocrine syndromes with small-cell lung cancer (not squamous), but in fact small-cell cancer does not produce hypercalcemia. Tumors causing HHM secrete PTH-related peptide (PTH-rP), which acts in a fashion similar to PTH. PTH-rP is present in small amounts in normal persons and is necessary for development of cartilage cells, mammary glands, hair follicles, and skin, and in fact appears to be the "parathyroid hormone" of the fetus. Patients with pathological PTH-rP secretion, however, have laboratory findings similar to patients with hyperparathyroidism: hypercalcemia with hypophosphatemia. Native PTH secretion is inhibited by hypercalcemia, so PTH levels are low.

Local osteolytic hypercalcemia (LOH) is a less common cause of tumor-associated hypercalcemia. This disorder is due to secretion substances called OAFs (osteoclast activating factors), not by direct tumor invasion by bone. Examples include breast cancer and multiple myeloma.

VITAMIN D-DEPENDENT HYPERCALCEMIA

Hypercalcemia may also occur if excess vitamin D is present. The manufacture of vitamin D is tightly regulated by feedback inhibition, so synthesis of the active metabolites (e.g. calcitriol) is usually shut off when ordinary vitamin D (e.g., from multivitamins) is ingested. Vitamin D toxicity may occur when high-potency pharmacologic preparations (e.g., ergocalciferol, dihydrotachysterol, calcitriol) are ingested.

Granulomatous diseases (such as tuberculosis, sarcoidosis, berylliosis, and leprosy) may also cause vitamin D–dependent hypercalcemia. The cells of these lesions may possess the enzyme necessary to convert more primitive vitamin D forms to calcitriol, resulting in hypercalcemia.

The treatment of vitamin D–dependent hypercalcemia obviously involves removal of the vitamin D source, if present. Treatment of the systemic diseases mentioned above is important. Glucocorticoids are a mainstay of treatment because they decrease calcium absorption from the intestine and result in a prompt decrease in calcium levels.

OTHER CAUSES

Some endocrine disorders also may cause hypercalcemia. Hyperthyroidism may lead to increased bone resorption of calcium. This hypercalcemia is usually mild, with few or no symptoms, and responds promptly to treatment. Persistence of hypercalcemia after treatment suggests another cause.

Adrenal insufficiency also may cause mild hypercalcemia. This condition is aggravated by the dehydration that normally occurs during adrenal insufficiency. Rehydration and steroid replacement promptly restore calcium levels to normal.

Milk-alkali syndrome may occur after the ingestion of large amounts of calcium (e.g., milk) and alkali (e.g., sodium bicarbonate), usually taken for a peptic ulcer or esophagitis. The metabolic alkalosis results in hypocalciuria and later, hypercalcemia. Renal failure often occurs. This disorder is uncommon today because of vastly improved treatments of peptic ulcer disease, and at one time was felt to be an extinct entity. It was much more common in the past, when ulcer patients drank whole bottles of milk along with boxes of baking soda ($NaHCO_3$). Recently, however, there has been increased use of calcium for prevention of osteoporosis. Some patients consume more than the prescribed amount of calcium, resulting in more cases of this syndrome in recent years.

HYPERCALCEMIC CRISIS

Hypercalcemic crisis is the end stage of hypercalcemia, and may lead to coma and death. Although any of the above conditions can cause it, it usually is associated with malignancy. Since these patients are usually severely dehydrated (calcium acts as an osmotic diuretic), the most important first step is rehydration with intravenous fluids. After rehydration has been established, loop diuretics (furosemide) promote calciuria, and are especially useful in those with renal failure.

Glucocorticoids are useful in the vitamin D–dependent hypercalcemias, hypercalcemia of adrenal insufficiency, and hypercalcemia associated with certain osteolytic tumors, but are of minimal use in other conditions. Humoral hypercalcemia of malignancy is best treated with an antiresorptive agent. These include the bisphosphonates (pamidronate and etidronate), which bind irreversibly to bone and prevent its resorption, the antibiotic plicamycin (mithramycin), and gallium nitrate. Salmon calcitonin has mild antiresorptive action and is useful in mild hypercalcemia. After calcium levels have returned to normal, treatment of the underlying disease is indicated.

HYPOCALCEMIA

Whereas hypercalcemia causes neuromuscular suppression, hypocalcemia results in neuromuscular excitability. Typical manifestations include paresthesias (numbness and tingling), hyperventilation, tetany, adrenergic symptoms (e.g., tachycardia, diaphoresis), seizures, Chvostek's and Trousseau's signs, QT interval prolongation, hypotension, refractory CHF, cardiomegaly, abnormalities in dental formation, gastrointestinal malabsorption, and cataracts.

Chvostek's and Trousseau's signs may be seen in those with hypocalcemia and latent tetany. Chvostek's sign is elicited by tapping the face in the area of the facial nerve. A positive response is spasm of the facial muscles on that side. Many normal persons have a slight Chvostek's sign. Trousseau's sign is elicited by inflating a blood pressure cuff around the arm between systolic and diastolic blood pressures. This is continued for several minutes, and the time to carpal spasm is noted, if positive.

Hypocalcemia may be caused by many conditions. Just as hypercalcemia can be caused by too much parathyroid hormone (PTH), hypocalcemia may occur if there is not enough. This condition is called hypoparathyroidism and the most common cause is inadvertent surgical damage or removal (e.g., from removal of the thyroid). It also may be present for no apparent reason (idiopathic). In addition to hypocalcemia, hyperphosphatemia may be present, since PTH normally promotes phosphorus excretion by the body.

Persons with hypoparathyroidism have low calcium levels, because PTH effects on bone and kidney are diminished. Hyperphosphatemia is present, since PTH normally causes phosphate excretion by the kidney. PTH levels are of course diminished.

The treatment of hypoparathyroidism is one example where the native hormone is not normally used as a replacement. This means that its effects on the two major sites—kidney and bone—are lost forever. Its third effect (that of enhancing calcitriol production) can be mimicked by administering calcitriol or other vitamin D analogs orally. With sufficient doses and dietary calcium supplementation, serum calcium levels return to normal.

Another condition similar to hypoparathyroidism occurs when the body is resistant to PTH action. This produces a clinical picture similar to hypoparathyroidism, except that the PTH levels are elevated. This syndrome is called pseudohypoparathyroidism (false hypoparathyroidism). In addition to the hypocalcemia and hyperphosphatemia, these patients often have some characteristic clinical features: short stature, obesity, short fourth metacarpals (brachydactyly), and mental retardation. The treatment of pseudohypoparathyroidism is similar to that of hypoparathyroidism (vitamin D analogs plus calcium supplementation).

You might ask if hypocalcemia can occur because of dietary deficiency. This is not likely, because the skeleton contains vast amounts of calcium, which is adequate to keep calcium levels normal (even in the face of dietary deficiency). The cost is, however, loss of bone, leading to osteoporosis.

A good way to help determine the etiology of hyper- or hypocalcemia is to plot the serum calcium concentration against the PTH level. This helps divide the values into four categories: low calcium, low PTH; low calcium, high PTH; high calcium, high PTH; and high calcium, low PTH.

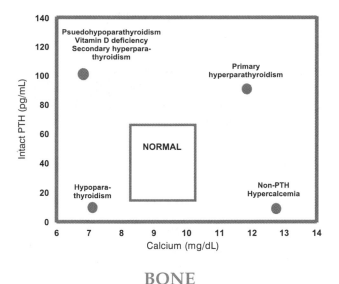

BONE

Bone provides rigid support and protection for extremities and body cavities containing vital organs, and provides effective levers for muscles. It serves as a large reservoir of ions (calcium, magnesium, and phosphorus). Without bone, we would simply be a large mass of organic protoplasm quivering on the floor. A marvel of engineering, it provides enormous support and strength while being relatively lightweight.

There are two major types of bone. Cortical or compact bone is found in tubular bones (e.g., radius, tibia). Trabecular or cancellous bone is found in the vertebrae and axial skeleton.

Bone is more than just a hard structure that supports our tissues; it is a living organ that is constantly being remodeled. It consists of a matrix (collagenous proteins which form the framework) and minerals (calcium salts laid over the matrix). The molecules in your femur today are not the same as three years ago. Normally, the amount resorbed equals the amount formed. Osteoblasts form new bone on the surface and synthesize new matrix (collagenous proteins). Osteocytes are merely osteoblasts after they are trapped in mineralized matrix. Osteoclasts are multinucleated giant cells involved in bone resorption.

OSTEOPOROSIS

Osteoporosis is the condition of a decreased quantity of bone (mineralization + matrix). It is a common medical disorder occurring in 10 million Americans. Osteoporosis causes more than 1.5 million fractures each year, including more than 300,000 hip fractures and 700,000 vertebral fractures. One in two women over the age of 50 and one in eight men over age 50 will have an osteoporosis-related fracture in their lifetime. The estimated national direct expenditure for hospital and nursing homes for fractures related to osteoporosis was $13.8 billion in 1995.

The pathogenesis of osteoporosis involves uncoupling of the normal balance between bone formation and resorption. The bone present is structurally normal. In normal health, the amount formed equals amount resorbed. In osteoporosis, either too much bone is resorbed (high turnover), or too little is formed (low turnover).

What are some risk factors for osteoporosis? Genetics obviously play a role; like most disorders, patients are more likely to have osteoporosis if they have a strong family history. Certain ethnic groups are more likely to develop osteoporosis. Traditionally, those of northern European and Asian descent are more likely to develop osteoporosis than other groups. Patients who are overweight are less likely to develop osteoporosis (at least one positive thing about being overweight!). Overweight persons may have increased bone mass compared to normal people because of the stress on the bones of carrying extra weight around. Cigarette smoking is a risk factor for osteoporosis as is excess alcohol consumption. Immobilization is another risk factor for osteoporosis. Patients who are bedridden for a long time eventually lose a great deal of bone mass. Space scientists discovered that astronauts in a weightless environment lost a tremendous amount of bone density unless they engaged in regular exercise aboard the spacecraft. Without adequate exercise an astronaut taking a one-year long trip to Mars would break his or her legs after stepping onto the Martian surface merely from the loss of bone mass during the trip.

The most frequent cause of osteoporosis in women is postmenopausal. Most bone loss occurs within the first 10 years after menopause or oophorectomy, and is a high turnover form of osteoporosis (estrogen deficiency enhances bone resorption). Not all postmenopausal patients develop osteoporosis—it is important to identify those patients at risk and treat with estrogen as soon as possible.

Corticosteroids are the most common cause of drug-induced osteoporosis, since they are used for many chronic diseases. Since they inhibit bone formation, this is a low turnover form of osteoporosis.

Osteoporosis is uncommon in men, because they start out with higher bone mass than women. Men with testosterone deficiency (hypogonadism) may develop osteoporosis.

Osteoporosis is a straightforward diagnosis for patients with obvious osteopenia on x-ray and pathologic fractures (e.g., compression fracture of the spine).

Plain x-ray, however, is usually a poor method of diagnosing osteoporosis, because a tremendous amount of bone must be lost before it can be detected. The test of choice is DEXA (dual-energy x-ray absorptiometry), which is noninvasive and easy to perform.

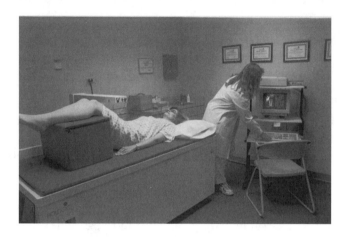

Bone density is typically measured in the lumbar spine and femoral neck, and plotted on a graph. The values are compared to others in his/her age group and to young adults. It has been found that fracture correlates best when compared to young adults (peak bone mass) than with others the same age. For example, a 95-year old woman with a bone density at the 75th percentile for her age still has significant risk of fracture since practically all persons this age have some osteopenia.

Bone density, like most human measurements, is normally distributed. Persons with a bone density greater than the 16th percentile (greater than one standard deviation below the mean) for young adults are said to have normal bone density. Those with bone density between –2.5 and –1.0 standard deviations below the mean have low bone mass or osteopenia. Those with a value less than 2.5 standard deviations below the mean (<2nd percentile) have osteoporosis. Just like not everyone is tall, not everyone has a high bone density; someone has to be below the mean. Risk of fracture is also relative, and patients with low bone densities may never

have fractures if they are sedentary. On the other hand, 300-pound pro-football linemen with very high bone densities routinely suffer fractures after smashing into each other on Sunday afternoons.

Laboratory studies of people with osteoporosis are typically normal. However, screening to exclude secondary causes should be considered in many patients to exclude metabolic disease.

TREATMENT OF OSTEOPOROSIS

There are many treatments for osteoporosis. In patients with hypogonadism, it is usually desirable to replace the sex steroids. In postmenopausal or oophorectomized women in whom it is not contraindicated (those with breast cancer or active thromboembolic disease), estrogen is the best treatment. It is much more effective if started soon after menopause or oophorectomy, since most bone is lost during the first five years after menopause or oophorectomy. Men with hypogonadism should receive androgen therapy.

Bisphosphonates (already discussed with treatment of hypercalcemia) are phosphate analogs that bind to bone, thus preventing resorption. They also stimulate bone formation to a mild degree. Alendronate and risedronate are oral bisphosphonates used for osteoporosis.

Salmon calcitonin also inhibits bone resorption and has an analgesic effect. It is available either as a subcutaneous form or as a nasal spray. Raloxifene is a synthetic estrogen receptor modulator (SERM) that may be given to certain patients who cannot tolerate estrogen or in whom estrogen is contraindicated (e.g., breast cancer survivors). It has the anti-resorptive properties of estrogen but no other hormonal effects, so it is not useful in preventing symptoms such as hot flashes. Calcium and vitamin D supplementation are recommended in all patients. Risks for osteoporosis (smoking, corticosteroids) should be reduced or eliminated if possible.

OSTEOMALACIA

Osteomalacia is another disorder of calcium metabolism that is biochemically distinct from osteoporosis. In osteoporosis, both calcification and organic matrix are deficient. In osteomalacia, the organic matrix is normal, but calcification is deficient. When osteomalacia occurs in children, it is called rickets.

Patients with osteomalacia commonly develop deformities caused by fractures in ribs, vertebrae, and long bones, and often have a "waddling gait" with muscle weakness and diffuse skeletal pain. A classic radiologic finding is the presence of a radiolucent band (called pseudofractures or Looser's zones), often in the long bones, metatarsals, pelvis, and scapula.

The etiology of osteomalacia is usually from vitamin D deficiency, which leads to hypocalcemia and hypophosphatemia. Less commonly, metabolic errors in calcium and/or phosphorus metabolism can cause this disorder. Drugs such as some anticonvulsants may interfere with vitamin D metabolism and cause osteomalacia. Serum calcidiol is typically low, and parathyroid hormone levels are increased if the patient has hypocalcemia. Alkaline phosphatase (a marker of bone formation) is usually elevated.

The treatment of osteomalacia includes vitamin D analogs (e.g., calcitriol), dietary calcium, and phosphate, which restore calcium and phosphorus levels to normal. Malabsorption also should be treated, if present. Tumor-associated osteomalacia is an interesting condition in which osteomalacia appears to be caused by some type of humoral factor secreted by the tumor. This disorder improves with treatment of the malignancy.

PAGET'S DISEASE OF BONE

Finally, let's discuss another type of disorder called Paget's disease, which is basically an error in bone remodeling. In normal bone, bone formation equals bone resorption at all sites. In Paget's disease, however, excessive resorption and formation occur at different sites, resulting in a disorganized mosaic of bone at affected sites. It is a common disorder, although many cases go undiagnosed because of the lack of symptoms.

Most patients are asymptomatic and discovered incidentally by x-ray, bone scan, or elevated alkaline phosphatase level. Few patients present with pain directly related to the pagetic process. Bowing deformities of the limbs can lead to pain, shortened limbs, and gait abnormalities. The normal side may be affected by abnormal weight bearing. Osteoarthritis is a common secondary complication, and it may be difficult to separate this from pagetic pain.

7 REPRODUCTIVE ENDOCRINOLOGY

REVIEW

Let's review what we learned in the last lecture. Calcium is an important ion in regulating many processes, including muscle contraction, transmission of impulses in the nervous system, and coagulation. It also is an important second messenger in hormone action. It is not under direct control by the pituitary gland or hypothalamus and is not a "classic" endocrine hormone since it is not secreted by a gland.

Calcium is bound to serum proteins such as albumin. Only the free or unbound (ionized) portion of calcium is biologically active. The major source of calcium is the skeleton, which contains over 99% of the body's calcium stores. The main regulator of calcium metabolism is parathyroid hormone, which is made by the parathyroid glands. Parathyroid hormone secretion increases when hypocalcemia occurs.

Another hormone important in calcium metabolism is vitamin D. This may be obtained from the diet but also can be produced by exposing the skin to the sun. The hormone calcitonin is a weak antagonist to PTH, and has no significance in humans.

Hypercalcemia may be caused by several disorders. Mild hypercalcemia is most commonly caused by primary hyperparathyroidism and has few symptoms. The only effective treatment for hyperparathyroidism at this time is surgery, although experimental oral treatments are being investigated. Severe hypercalcemia is often brought about by malignancy, and may cause neuromuscular suppressibility, psychosis, coma, and even death. Most commonly, malignancies produce hypercalcemia by secreting a substance called parathyroid hormone related protein (PTH-rP). Other tumors may produce hypercalcemia by secreting factors that dissolve bone (osteoclast activating factors). Too much vitamin D can also cause hypercalcemia. This usually occurs when high-potency pharmacologic preparations are ingested.

The treatment of hypercalcemia depends on the etiology. Hyperparathyroidism is normally treated by surgery. Care of malignancy-associated hypercalcemia includes treatment of the tumor and administration of anti-resorptive agents, such as pamidronate.

Hypocalcemia causes neuromuscular excitability and may result in muscular spasms and seizures. One cause of hypercalcemia is hypoparathyroidism, in which the body produces too little parathyroid hormone. The treatment of hypoparathyroidism involves administration of potent vitamin D analogs, since synthetic PTH is not widely available at this time for administration. Pseudohypoparathyroidism is another disorder that results from tissue resistance to PTH. These patients often have characteristic clinical features and have elevated PTH levels because of hormone resistance.

Bone is a rigid support for extremities, helps provide levers for locomotion and protection for vital organs, and also serves as a large reservoir for calcium and other ions. It is a living organism constantly being remodeled. Osteoporosis results when the amount of bone that is made is less than the amount that is resorbed. The most common cause of osteoporosis is hypogonadism in women, secondary to menopause or oophorectomy. Estrogen helps decrease the risk of osteoporosis. Another common cause of osteoporosis is exposure to large amounts of glucocorticoids. Osteoporosis is best diagnosed with a special x-ray study called DEXA. Treatments for osteoporosis include estrogen, calcium supplementation, bisphosphonates, calcitonin, and estrogen-like drugs such as raloxifene.

AN INTRODUCTION TO REPRODUCTIVE ENDOCRINOLOGY

Reproduction is vital to the continued survival of any organism. In addition to propagation of the species, hormones secreted by the sex organs are important in other bodily processes. For example, sex steroids are necessary for normal bone metabolism. This lecture deals with the development and endocrine function of the reproductive systems in men and women.

In our football team analogy, think of the reproductive system as the scouts who look for new talent for the draft. If the team did not draft new players, the old players would retire and the team would cease to exist. The new players ensure that a vital core of players is present at all times.

REGULATION OF TESTICULAR FUNCTION

The testes contain two important cell types. Sertoli cells are the site of spermatogenesis, and are stimulated by the pituitary hormone follicle-stimulating hormone (FSH). The other cell of interest is the Leydig cell, the site of testosterone synthesis; the stimulus for this is luteinizing hormone (LH). As with most feedback loops, the trophic hormone (LH) is inhibited by the end product (testosterone) and high levels result in low LH levels. Other minor androgens (e.g., dehydroepiandrosterone, androstenedione) are also present, but testosterone is the major androgen of the reproductive system. A small proportion of testosterone in males originates in the adrenal cortex.

The hypothalamic hormone GnRH (gonadotropinhormone releasing hormone), when secreted in a pulsatile fashion (every 90 minutes), stimulates gonadotropin (FSH and LH). If given continuously, GnRH actually results in paradoxical inhibition of gonadotropin secretion.

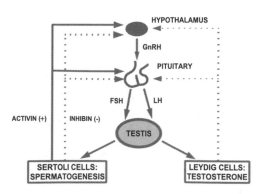

OVARIAN CYCLE REGULATION

The reproductive unit of the female is the ovum, which contains theca and granulosa cells. Many follicles (groups of ova) develop in the ovary, but only one is destined to develop fully, and the others degenerate. The two main female sex steroids are estradiol and progesterone. Approximately 50% of testosterone in women originates in the ovaries, and the rest comes from the adrenal cortex and aromatization (conversion) of other steroids in peripheral tissues (e.g., fat). Estradiol is synthesized in several steps. Initially, androgenic precursors (testosterone and androstenedione) are made in the theca interna cells under the influence of luteinizing hormone (LH). The androgens then are aromatized to estradiol and estrone in the granulosa cells under the influence of follicle-stimulating hormone (FSH). This unique process is called the two-cell concept of ovarian steroid synthesis.

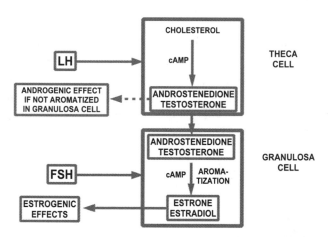

WITHOUT FSH, ANDROGEN SECRETION PREDOMINATES

The ovarian cycle may be divided into follicular (proliferative) and luteal (secretory) phases. Like in the male, pulsatile secretion of hypothalamic GnRH facilitates secretion of the gonadotropins LH and FSH. Early in the follicular phase, FSH secretion predominates, which increases the number of follicles and granulosa cells. Only one of many follicles is destined to become "ripe" for ovulation. LH secretion then increases, leading to theca cell proliferation. As estradiol concentrations increase, FSH secretion decreases. During this phase, the endometrium thickens and grows in length, mucus is secreted from the cervix, and maturation of the vaginal epithelium occurs (due to the effects of estrogens). Most follicles regress as the FSH secretion diminishes, but hopefully one will have enough receptors to remain viable. This is the one selected to ovulate.

In the viable follicle, estradiol concentrations increase, and although estrogen normally inhibits LH production, in this instance there is a paradoxical switch from negative to positive feedback, resulting in a pituitary LH surge. This culminates in ovulation, and the ovum is expelled from the ovary.

Then, the granulosa cells also acquire LH receptors and begin to secrete progesterone (the luteal phase), with the formation of the corpus luteum. Progesterone concentrations continue to increase, the glands become longer and edematous, and estradiol levels remain high. If the ovum is not fertilized, involution of the corpus luteum (luteolysis) occurs, and the endometrium is sloughed away (menstruation).

If the ovum is fertilized, the fetoplacental unit begins secreting the glycoprotein hormone β-hCG (human chorionic gonadotropin). This maintains the hormonal secretion of the corpus luteum. (Pregnancy tests detect hCG, either in the blood or the urine.) The elevated estrogen levels suppress FSH, preventing further ovulation.

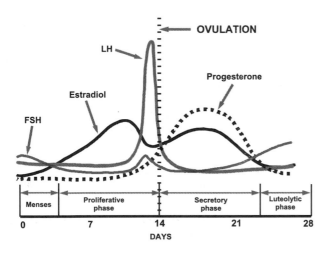

GONADAL DIFFERENTIATION

The embryonic gonads are indistinguishable until about six weeks. If a Y chromosome is present (male), a special protein called testis-determining factor is secreted, and the embryonic gonad becomes a testis. If there is no Y chromosome (female), an ovary develops. This is the traditional "female by default" hypothesis.

The presence or absence of a testis also determines which internal structures develop. The functional Sertoli cells of the testis secrete a hormone called müllerian inhibitory factor (MIF), which causes the müllerian (female) structures (uterus, uterine tubes, cervix, and upper third of the vagina) to disappear. The wolffian (male) structures (epididymis, vas deferens, seminal vesicles, and ejaculatory ducts) then develop in this case. If there is no testis, MIF is not secreted and the müllerian structures develop while the wolffian structures become vestigial remnants.

The type of external genitalia also is determined by (you guessed it) the presence or absence of a functional testis. Up to about eight weeks, the external genitalia may differentiate into those of either sex. A functional testis secretes small amounts of testosterone, and causes the differentiation into male external genitalia. In the absence of a testis, female external genitalia develop.

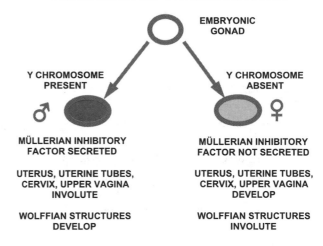

EFFECTS OF SEX STEROIDS

Testosterone results in differentiation of the internal and external male genital system and growth of the scrotum, epididymis, vas deferens, seminal vesicles, prostate, and penis. It also results in skeletal muscle, laryngeal, and long bone growth in both sexes. Estradiol causes maturation of the vagina, uterus, and uterine tubes in females at puberty. It also alters the distribution and type of body fat to a more female or "gynecoid" type found on the hips, buttocks, and thighs. Typical male or "android" fat is more central (e.g., a beer belly) and predominantly in the abdomen.

PUBERTY

The newborn infant possesses all the machinery necessary to go into puberty. Fortunately for society, this does not normally happen until the adolescent years, because the hypothalamic-pituitary axis (HPA) is held in check by potent inhibitory mechanisms. In the prepubertal child, very small circulating amounts of sex steroids inhibit gonadotropin secretion.

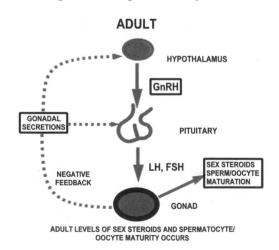

PRE-PUBERTY

LOW GONADAL STEROID LEVELS RESULT DUE TO SENSITIVITY
OF HYPOTHALAMUS TO VERY LOW CIRCULATING LEVELS

At puberty the inhibition decreases, and the gonadotropin-hormone releasing hormone (GnRH) begins secreting in a pulsatile fashion—every 90 minutes. This results in increased gonadotropin secretion and gonadal growth. The onset of gonadal stimulation is termed gonadarche. The pulsatile secretion of GnRH is very important—if it is given continuously, LH and FSH secretion is paradoxically suppressed. Eventually, sex steroid levels remain at adult levels, where they remain throughout the reproductive years.

ADULT

ADULT LEVELS OF SEX STEROIDS AND SPERMATOCYTE/
OOCYTE MATURITY OCCURS

Ninety-nine percent of boys and girls will begin puberty between ages 9 and 14 and ages 8 and 13, respectively. Those who do not have onset of puberty by age 13 (♀) or 14 (♂) are said to have delayed puberty. Those with onset of puberty before age 8 (♀) or 9 (♂) are said to have precocious puberty.

Boys and girls start with relatively equal lean body mass. Due to the effects of testosterone, males end up on average with 1.5 times as much muscle mass and 0.5 times as much fat as females. There is, of course, individual variation (female bodybuilders have more muscle mass and less fat than many males). Increasing androgen secretion (males and females) results in deepening voice and acne. Sex steroids and growth hormone result in increased bone density, with peak values occurring in the mid-twenties.

Sex steroids result in an initial increase (spurt) in growth velocity, but eventually result in closing of the epiphyseal plates of long bones and cessation of growth. Since puberty begins earlier in girls than boys, the epiphyseal plates close sooner, and they typically are shorter than boys, other things being equal.

The Tanner stages refer to specific developmental milestones that occur in puberty. The stages are numbered 1 through 5: 1 is prepubertal, 5 is adult development. Girls typically start puberty sooner, with the initial sign of puberty in a girl being breast budding. The growth spurt starts earlier in girls, and ends sooner. The first physical sign of puberty in a boy is testicular enlargement.

Adrenarche (also called pubarche) is another milestone of puberty and heralds the onset of adrenal androgen secretion. It is responsible for a large proportion of androgen secretion in girls. It is responsible for much of the terminal (dark, pigmented) hair in the axillary and pubic areas, and development of sweat glands in those areas (resulting in the characteristic pungent adult body odor). Terminal hair is coarse, pigmented, and has a greater potential for growth than vellus (fine, nonpigmented, "peach fuzz") hair. Terminal hair occurs on the scalp, eyebrows, and to varying degrees, on the body depending on the amount of circulating androgens and genetic differences in hair sensitivity. Vellus hair transforms into terminal hair given sufficient androgen concentrations. This accounts for the typical heavy terminal hair growth (face, chest, and extremities) seen in males. Pubic and axillary hair appears to require lower androgen concentrations than other hair for transformation. This results in increased testosterone secretion and development of pubic and axillary hair and acne.

Some terminal hair, such as on the scalp, has a tendency to de-differentiate into vellus hair under the influence of testosterone. This is what happens in men with male pattern baldness. Not all males develop this; the susceptibility appears to be genetically transmitted and is manifested as increased sensitivity of scalp hair to testosterone. Some women also develop male pattern baldness.

DELAYED PUBERTY

Another common presenting complaint is delayed puberty. This is defined as the absence of any pubertal development in a boy of 14 or girl of 13. The most common cause is constitutional delay, in which the child is destined to develop normally but is simply delayed a few years. These persons do eventually go through puberty normally and reach a height appropriate for their genetic predispositions. There is usually a positive family history in parents and siblings. It is important to distinguish those with constitutional delay from those with organic disease (e.g., growth hormone deficiency).

Growth charts in children with constitutional delay demonstrate early short stature, with eventual increase into the normal range.

Another test, called a bone age (BA) study, is also useful. This test compares an x-ray of the wrist bones to a set of normal x-rays. Bones characteristically change with age, until the epiphyses fuse. Normally, bone age (BA) equals chronologic age (CA) during the developmental years. In those with delayed puberty, the full effect of sex steroids has not been realized, and the bone age is delayed (BA<CA). Children with early onset (precocious) puberty have BA>CA. BA therefore can be used to estimate a child's remaining growth.

Pathological causes of delayed puberty include hypopituitarism (due to growth hormone and/or gonadotropin deficiency), hypothyroidism, hypogonadism, and chromosomal abnormalities.

PRECOCIOUS PUBERTY

Precocious puberty (PP) is defined as the onset of secondary sexual development in a girl before age 8 or a boy before age 9. Most commonly, PP is central (complete or "true"), meaning that puberty occurs via premature activation of the hypothalamic-pituitary axis (HPA). It is called true because it occurs by the same mechanism as normal puberty, except at an earlier age. Peripheral ("incomplete") PP is caused by abnormal gonadotropin and/or sex steroid secretion, rather than premature activation of the HPA.

As we discussed earlier, the potential for pubertal development is present at birth, but is held in check by strong inhibitory mechanisms. If these are disturbed, puberty commences and sexual maturation and fertility are achieved. Any central nervous system lesion that disrupts the normal inhibitory responses can cause this (e.g., hydrocephalus and central nervous system tumors). Central PP may also be "idiopathic," where no obvious cause may be found.

Incomplete or peripheral PP may be caused by any condition that results in increased gonadotropin and/or sex steroid secretion (exogenous steroids, premature adrenarche, congenital adrenal hyperplasia, steroid-secreting adrenal tumors, steroid-secreting ovarian/testicular tumors, and gonadotropin-secreting tumors).

In all forms of PP, since sex steroid secretion occurs at an early age, premature skeletal growth and epiphyseal closure occurs, resulting in early tall stature but eventual short stature. Early sexual development may also be psychologically devastating to the child.

Just like constitutional delayed puberty, a child may have constitutional early puberty. There is typically a family history of such and these children are often overweight. These children are large for their age but stop growing early at a normal adult height. As seen here, the growth curve appears normal but is shifted to the left two or three years (the opposite of constitutional delay).

The treatment for central PP is to somehow "shut off" the hypothalamic-pituitary axis (HPA). The best way to accomplish this is to administer long-lasting GnRH analogs such as leuprolide, which cause paradoxical gonadotropin suppression when given continuously (remember that it only stimulates the pituitary when secreted in pulsatile fashion). The child is given these drugs until the agent is withdrawn at the appropriate age, and the child goes through puberty normally.

Treatment for peripheral PP involves locating the site of steroid excess (e.g., tumor, congenital adrenal enzyme defect) and treating it (e.g., surgical removal, medical therapy).

HYPOGONADISM

Hypogonadism is the condition of sex steroid deficiency. It may be primary (due to a gonadal defect). This is also termed hypergonadotropic hypogonadism because gonadotropin levels (from the pituitary gland) are elevated. Secondary (lack of gonadotropin secretion) or tertiary (lack of GnRH) forms of hypogonadism are called hypogonadotropic.

A famous drawing by Leonardo da Vinci depicts a man with his hands stretched out and fitting perfectly into a square box. In a normal person, therefore, arm span roughly equals height, and the ratio of the upper to the lower body segment is approximately one. In hypogonadal states, however, body proportions become abnormal. Sex steroids initially cause an acceleration of bone age during the growth spurt. Although all long bones have a finite potential for growth, sex steroids eventually hasten closure of the epiphyses and cessation of linear growth. Sex steroid secretion peaks a bit earlier in girls than boys, resulting in girls being initially taller than boys (due to estrogen-induced acceleration of bone age early on) and stopping growth sooner (because of earlier epiphyseal fusion). With inadequate sex steroid secretion, bone age may be delayed a bit. However, they do continue to grow under the influence of growth hormone, and because of the lack of effect on epiphyseal closure, the long bones grow longer than they should, leading to disproportionately long arms and legs. **This person no longer fits inside the square, as the arms are too long. The lower body segment is also longer than the upper body segment.** These abnormalities are termed hypogonadal or eunuchoidal body proportions.

In an adult with hypogonadism, measuring body proportions is one way to tell whether or not the problem began prior to or after puberty; if the proportions are normal, the defect occurred in adulthood, after normal growth had ceased.

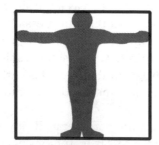

**NORMAL BODY PROPORTIONS
ARM SPAN = HEIGHT
UPPER = LOWER BODY SEGMENT**

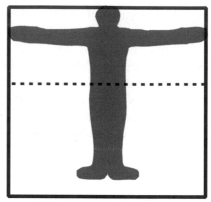

**HYPOGONADAL OR EUNUCHOIDAL PROPORTIONS
ARM SPAN > HEIGHT
UPPER < LOWER BODY SEGMENT**

We all know that women in middle age go through an abrupt decline in ovarian function called menopause. Some have proposed a similar phenomenon in males, called "andropause," in which male hormone levels abruptly decline, but there is little evidence to suggest such a phenomenon. Most males retain sexual function and fertility well into the sixth and seventh decades of life. Testosterone levels decline approximately 1 to 2 percent each year after age 30.

HYPOGONADOTROPIC HYPOGONADISM

This type of hypogonadism is caused by a defect in either GnRH (hypothalamus) or gonadotropin (LH and FSH) secretion. The most common cause is Kallmann's syndrome, a disorder of GnRH secretion associated with anosmia (inability to smell). **Other midline defects, such as a cleft palate, may be seen. It is much more common in males. The interesting thing about this syndrome is that the patients do not realize they cannot smell until you test them,** because they do not understand what smell is—it is like asking a congenitally blind person to describe color. Sense of smell can be qualitatively measured with any number of things commonly available at a supermarket: coffee, wintergreen, fruit extract, etc.

Hypogonadotropic hypogonadism may also be caused by any condition that disrupts pituitary function (e.g., hypopituitarism, hypothalamic destruction).

The treatment of hypogonadotropic hypogonadism depends on the desired result. If fertility is not desired, testosterone (male) or estrogen (female) replacement is given. If fertility is desired, gonadal stimulation can be induced by administration of gonadotropins. The glycoprotein β-hCG (human chorionic gonadotropin) has LH-like activity and is given along with FSH. Fertility can be induced in both sexes, but is more difficult in women because of the greater complexity of the female reproductive cycle. Alternatively, GnRH may be given in pulsatile fashion by a subcutaneous infusion pump, which induces LH and FSH secretion by the pituitary. It must be given in pulses every 90 minutes, since continuous therapy results in paradoxical suppression of the pituitary.

HYPERGONADOTROPIC HYPOGONADISM

Hypergonadotropic hypogonadism is due to a primary gonadal defect, and results in high gonadotropin levels (since the hypothalamus and pituitary function normally). In males, the most common cause is a chromosomal abnormality called Klinefelter's syndrome, occurring in 1 in 1000 males. In females, the most common cause is Turner's syndrome, with an incidence of 1 in 3000 girls. Other causes are less common and include congenital anorchia, cryptorchidism, gonadal damage (chemotherapy, radiation therapy), gonadectomy, and mumps orchitis.

Klinefelter's syndrome males typically have a 47, XXY cell karyotype (46, XY is normal). Testes are usually small and hard, and do not function properly. Since testosterone levels are deficient during adolescence, "eunuchoidal" proportions develop. Gynecomastia (male breast enlargement) is common, and these individuals have a higher incidence of breast carcinoma. Behavioral problems are common, although mental retardation is rare.

Turner's syndrome is the most common cause of primary amenorrhea in girls and is associated with the absence of an X chromosome (45, X). Intelligence is usually normal. The characteristic physical abnormalities may include short stature, webbed neck, congenital heart or kidney abnormalities, coarctation of the aorta, cubitus valgus, and other associated endocrine diseases (e.g. hypothyroidism and diabetes mellitus).

Treatment of hypergonadotropic hypogonadism consists of giving replacement steroids (estrogen or testosterone). Human growth hormone (GH) therapy also improves short stature in girls with Turner's syndrome.

Testosterone Replacement

Testosterone is well absorbed by the intestine, but is virtually useless because it is rapidly degraded in the liver by something called the first-pass effect. Testosterone may be combined with an ester, producing a long-lasting compound that may be given intramuscularly. These testosterone esters are generally given every two weeks to one month. Transdermal testosterone is available, and is administered as a once-daily patch. A newly available gel preparation of testosterone can be applied to the skin once daily. Oral derivatives of testosterone that resist hepatic degradation are available. These compounds have been shown to cause liver damage and their use is not routinely recommended. Androgens carry a high potential for abuse and unfortunately have been used by some strength athletes, sometimes in doses 100 to 1000 times normal. Abuse of these drugs causes a variety of psychological and physiological problems. Illicit use of androgens is illegal in the United States.

Estrogen Replacement

Like testosterone, estradiol is well absorbed orally but rapidly degraded by the first-pass phenomenon. Micronized estradiol, however, produces satisfactory plasma levels. Conjugated estrogens have high bioavailability and are prepared from the urine of pregnant mares. Other compounds include esterified estrogens, estropipate, and ethinyl estradiol.

Women without a uterus may take continuous estrogen alone. Synthetic progestin (medroxyprogesterone) should be given to women who still have a uterus. One method is administering the estrogen for the first part of the month and adding progestin to the last week of the month, with withdrawal of both drugs for several days. This results in withdrawal menses similar to that of natural menses. This ensures that the uterine lining is sloughed each month, since unopposed estrogen stimulation leads to endometrial buildup, which can result in endometrial carcinoma. Another method is administering the estrogen and progestin continuously. This also decreases endometrial buildup and results in less bleeding than treatment with intermittent therapy.

Estrogen can also be given transdermally. The lipid-lowering effect is less when administered transdermally, since less estrogen passes through the liver (the site of lipoprotein synthesis). Those with a uterus are also given continuous progestin.

Estrogen should not be given to women with a history of breast cancer, as estrogen may stimulate tumor growth. Estrogen administration also results in a very small increase in breast cancer, so women with a strong family history may not wish to take it, although this is not an absolute contraindication. Estrogen should be avoided in those with active thromboembolic disease (e.g., recent pulmonary embolism on anticoagulant therapy) or those with the common Leiden factor V mutation (resistance to activated protein C), which predisposes patients to thromboembolism.

Selective estrogen receptor modulators (SERMs), such as raloxifene, appear to have protective effects against osteoporosis. These drugs do not help with vasomotor flashes, however. Like estrogen, they appear to increase the incidence of thromboembolism in susceptible individuals.

GYNECOMASTIA

Gynecomastia is the presence of abnormal breast enlargement in the male. It may occur whenever there is a decrease in the androgen:estrogen (A:E) ratio. This may happen with either androgen deficiency or estrogen excess. The most common cause is pubertal gynecomastia. Early in puberty, testicular steroidogenesis favors estrogen secretion. As puberty progresses, steroid synthesis favors androgen production, and pubertal gynecomastia disappears in most cases.

Obese boys also tend to have higher estrogen levels due to the peripheral conversion of androgen to estrogen in fat; their incidence of gynecomastia is higher. One must distinguish lipomastia (increased fat in the breast area) from true gynecomastia, since often the large breast appearance is simply fat.

Hypogonadism may obviously cause gynecomastia by decreasing the A:E ratio. It is very common in Klinefelter's syndrome. Adults may develop gynecomastia if hypogonadism occurs (e.g., men undergoing orchiectomy for prostate cancer). Many commonly used medications interfere with androgen production and may cause gynecomastia. Marijuana has an LH-like effect and may produce gynecomastia—just one more reason not to use it!

Steroid-producing (adrenal, testis) or β-hCG-producing (testis, lung) neoplasms can cause gynecomastia. Acromegaly results in soft tissue growth and can be another cause. It may also be associated with hypogonadism and/or hyperprolactinemia.

Pubertal gynecomastia is typically self-limited, and underlying disorders (e.g., hypogonadism, germ cell tumors) should be treated. In severe cases, a reduction mammoplasty should be considered. Patients with Klinefelter's syndrome have a higher incidence of breast carcinoma and should be checked regularly.

PRIMARY AMENORRHEA

Amenorrhea is the absence of menses. It is classified as primary (menses have never occurred) or secondary (menses have occurred before but have now stopped).

The most common cause of primary amenorrhea is Turner's syndrome. Müllerian agenesis is another common cause of primary amenorrhea. As the name implies, it is associated with absent müllerian structures. Since there is no uterus, menses cannot occur. The ovaries are normal and hence secondary sex characteristics are normal. Testicular feminization (discussed below) is also a relatively common cause of primary amenorrhea.

SECONDARY AMENORRHEA

Secondary amenorrhea is a condition in which menses have occurred previously but have stopped. In young women, the most common cause is anovulation. Polycystic ovary syndrome, to be discussed in detail later, is a common cause of anovulation in reproductive-age females. In older women, primary ovarian failure (menopause) is most likely. Other causes include hypothalamic amenorrhea, hypopituitarism, and hyperprolactinemia. Uterine outflow tract obstruction may cause secondary amenorrhea. In this case, the ovaries function normally, but menses cannot occur since menstrual outflow is blocked.

EVALUATION OF AMENORRHEA

The first goal is to determine if the ovaries are producing estrogen. Although estrogen levels can be measured, a simpler method of determining adequate estrogenization is a progestin challenge. In this test, a synthetic progesterone derivative (medroxyprogesterone) is given for several days. If adequate estrogenization has occurred, the menstrual lining is primed and will be sloughed off several days after administration of progestin. If withdrawal bleeding occurs after the progestin has been given for several days, this confirms adequate estrogenization and means that the amenorrhea is due to inadequate progesterone secretion (anovulation). If there is no withdrawal bleeding after progestin, a combination of estrogen and progestin is given. If withdrawal bleeding occurs, it suggests inadequate estrogenization (e.g., ovarian failure, hypothalamic amenorrhea). If there is no bleeding with combination therapy, there is either a mechanical outflow obstruction or no uterus present.

Hypothalamic amenorrhea is a functional abnormality in GnRH secretion resulting in low gonadotropin levels and secondary amenorrhea. It is common in young women with increased psychological stress (e.g., going away to college, breaking up with a boyfriend, starting a new job). It typically is a self-limited disorder. Other causes of hypogonadotropic amenorrhea include hypopituitarism and hyperprolactinemia.

CONSEQUENCES OF ESTROGEN DEFICIENCY IN WOMEN

Early estrogen deficiency leads to vaginal atrophy and dyspareunia (painful intercourse). A decrease in estrogen levels leads to stimulation of central thermoregulatory centers, with resultant vasomotor or hot flashes. The mechanism is unknown. Women who have a sudden decrease in estrogen (e.g., after oophorectomy) experience hot flashes to a greater degree than those with a slower decrease (e.g., natural menopause).

In the long term, estrogen deficiency may cause decreased bone mass and osteoporosis. This is a "high-turnover" form of osteoporosis, and most of the bone is lost within the first 10 to 15 years after menopause. It is therefore most beneficial to replace estrogen as soon as possible after menopause.

Estrogen also has beneficial cardiovascular effects, including increase in HDL cholesterol and decrease in LDL cholesterol. Estrogen deficiency leads to increase in android (central) obesity, which is more atherogenic than gynecoid obesity. Menopausal women who do not receive hormone replacement lose these beneficial effects.

HIRSUTISM

Hirsutism refers to the condition of excess terminal (pigmented) hair in women. Let us review the physiology of hair growth. Vellus hair is soft, fine, and nonpigmented, and transforms into terminal (coarse, pigmented) hair after stimulation by androgen. Terminal hair is androgen-dependent, except on the scalp and eyebrows. In these areas, androgens have the opposite effect. In many men, the terminal hair on the scalp is sensitive to androgen, causing reverse transformation to vellus hair (male pattern baldness). Male pattern baldness can also occur in women if androgen levels and/or hair sensitivity to androgen is high enough.

Women normally have terminal hair only on the scalp, eyebrows, and "adrenarchal" areas (axilla, pubic area). There is a marked genetic difference in amount of terminal hair expressed due to variability in androgen sensitivity; androgen levels are similar among all ethnic groups. The goal is to rule out serious underlying disease.

One must distinguish hirsutism (presence of excess terminal hair) from virilization (development of other masculine qualities such as increased muscle mass, deepening of the voice, and baldness). Virilization is much more suggestive of endocrine disease than simple hirsutism.

Most cases of hirsutism result from increased sensitivity to normal amounts of androgen (familial or idiopathic hirsutism). Some ethnic groups simply manifest more body hair than others, although actual androgen levels are similar. Any endocrine disorder resulting in an increased androgen-to-estrogen ratio may cause hirsutism, including virilizing adrenal and/or ovarian tumors, congenital adrenal hyperplasia, and polycystic ovary syndrome.

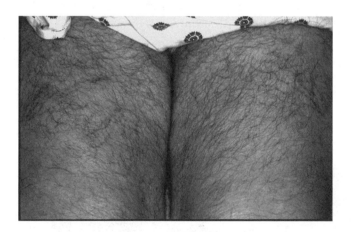

The treatment of hirsutism includes treatment of underlying disorders, if present. Many drugs are useful in the treatment of hirsutism. One class of drugs, the antiandrogens, blocks the effect of testosterone on its receptor; the most commonly used is the drug spironolactone. Oral contraceptives decrease the androgen to estrogen ratio by increasing estrogen levels. DHT production is held back by 5α-reductase inhibitors (e.g., finasteride), with reduction in terminal hair. All these drugs can have adverse effects on a fetus, therefore be certain that the woman is not pregnant. A new topical drug, eflornithine, inhibits ornithine decarboxylase, an enzyme necessary for hair follicle development.

Cosmetic treatments for hirsutism include simply shaving or bleaching the hair. Removal of hair (epilation) can be accomplished by several methods. Electrolysis utilizes an electric current that permanently destroys the hair follicle, and many treatments may be required. Laser epilation has also shown promise as a treatment for hirsutism. Waxing, although commonly employed in this country, may actually cause increased irritation and worsen the problem if used repeatedly.

POLYCYSTIC OVARY SYNDROME (PCOS)

PCOS is a common disorder of chronic anovulation leading to increased estrogen production and infertility. To understand this disorder, remember the two-cell concept of steroidogenesis we discussed earlier. LH (luteinizing hormone) primarily stimulates the theca cells, which synthesize androgen from cholesterol. Androgens, in turn, are aromatized to estrogen in the granulosa cells under the influence of FSH (follicle-stimulating hormone).

Women with PCO are sort of stuck in a time warp at the middle of the reproductive cycle—their ovaries are trying desperately to ovulate in order to try and break the vicious cycle. Without ovulation, FSH levels are lower and androgen secretion predominates as a result. Instead, the increased LH levels lead to even more androgen production. Until this cycle is broken, the problem continues.

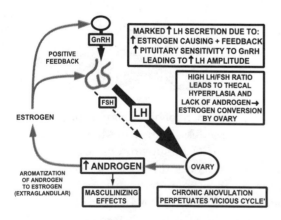

The characteristic woman with PCOS has chronic anovulation, "android" obesity, hyperinsulinism,

and hyperandrogenism. These components occur in varying degrees: not all women are obese, for example. Some have only minimal hirsutism, whereas in many it is quite severe.

Android obesity often results in hyperinsulinemia (insulin resistance) due to defective insulin receptor action and may lead to glucose intolerance and type 2 diabetes mellitus. Hyperinsulinemia, in turn, may increase androgen production, worsening the problem. Hyperandrogenism may then impair insulin action, leading to another vicious cycle.

Android fat is also metabolically active in aromatizing estrogen to androgen, and this obesity also plays a role. Hyperandrogenism itself can impair insulin action, which perpetuates the vicious cycle so predominant in PCOS.

The treatment of PCOS depends on the desired result. If the woman wants to have children, ovulation must be induced. This is typically performed with the estrogen agonist clomiphene citrate. This compound effectively inhibits the effects of stronger estrogens and permits gonadotropins to be secreted normally, allowing for ovulation. Other agents such as FSH may be used if this fails. Insulin-sensitizing drugs such as metformin and the thiazolidinediones (TZDs) theoretically would improve symptoms by decreasing insulin resistance. They have been used in patients with severe insulin resistance who have not responded to other therapies.

If fertility is not desired, a progestin may simply be given at the end of the month to induce withdrawal bleeding. This is necessary because the endometrium is hyperplastic and is at higher risk for transforming into endometrial carcinoma if not sloughed regularly. Hirsutism may be treated with the methods above. Weight loss may decrease hyperinsulinism and improve symptoms in obese women.

HERMAPHRODISM AND PSEUDOHERMAPHRODISM

Hermaphroditos, a character of ancient Greek mythology, was the son of Hermes and Aphrodite. The gods joined his body with that of a nymph who loved him, forming a single being who was both male and female—Hermaphrodite. The term hermaphrodism has been applied to many intersex conditions, but true hermaphrodism is an extremely rare condition in which both ovarian and testicular tissues are found in the same individual. Pseudohermaphroditism is a more common condition in which the phenotype (appearance) is opposite to that of the genetic sex; e.g., a female pseudohermaphrodite has a 46, XX (female) karyotype but appears male. A male pseudohermaphrodite appears female but has a 46, XY (male) karyotype. The most common cause in females is the 21-hydroxylase variant of congenital adrenal hyperplasia, which we discussed in Lecture 4. Causes in males include the feminizing forms of congenital adrenal hyperplasia and testicular feminization.

The differentiation of external and internal genitalia is highly variable, and most often ambiguous external genitalia are present.

Testicular feminization is one of the most interesting endocrine disorders and is a relatively common cause of primary amenorrhea and male pseudohermaphrodism in girls. These females are in fact genetic males (46, XY) who lack testosterone receptors, resulting in end-organ insensitivity to androgen, resulting in a hormone resistance syndrome. Since testosterone has no effect, wolffian (male) structures are absent, and müllerian (female) structures (uterus, uterine tubes, upper vagina) are absent, since the testes make müllerian inhibitory factor. In the complete form, total lack of masculinization occurs. They typically look so normal that no endocrine disorder is suspected until primary amenorrhea is discovered. A female hurdler with complete testicular feminization was in fact disqualified many years ago from the Olympics because of a 46, XY karyotype, despite the fact that she appeared to be a normal female and the disorder confers no competitive advantage. Girls with complete testicular feminization have only vellus hairs, except on the scalp and eyebrows. Because of decreased androgen effect, they may not suffer from acne and their voices may be higher-pitched than normal girls. They may lead normal lives as females (except for the inability to reproduce, of course).

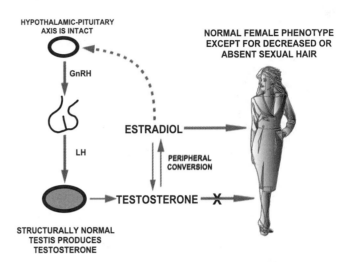

You may wonder how adequate estrogen is produced since these individuals lack ovaries. Testosterone of testicular origin is aromatized to estradiol in the peripheral compartment (fat). Levels are thus in the normal female range.

These girls have a normal female appearance and therefore are raised as such. They should always be referred to as female since this is their phenotypic appearance, and no reference should be made to their genetic karyotype. To tell these girls that they are really male is inappropriate, serves no logical purpose, and may cause significant psychological problems. The undescended (cryptorchid) testes are at higher risk for malignancy and should be removed at adulthood. Supplemental estrogen must then be given, as the source of estrogen will be gone. Since there is no uterus, menses cannot occur. Only the lower portion of the vagina is present, and ends in a blind pouch. Usually, a vagina long enough to permit intercourse is achievable by slowly introducing larger forms to stretch it. In severe cases, reconstructive surgery may be required.

8

LIPID DISORDERS

REVIEW

In the last lecture we learned about the function of the reproductive system. The testes contain two major cell types. The first are the Sertoli cells (the site of spermatogenesis), which are under the influence of follicle-stimulating hormone; they are the site of spermatogenesis. The Leydig cells are under the influence of luteinizing hormone and secrete testosterone. Under the pulsatile secretion of the hypothalamic hormone GnRH, the pituitary produces appropriate levels of FSH and LH. If GnRH is given continuously, however, a paradoxical decrease in gonadotropin secretion occurs.

Control of the ovary is more complex. The reproductive unit of the female is the ovum, which contains both theca and granulosa cells. Many follicles develop in the ovary while only one is destined to develop fully.

The ovarian cycle is divided into follicular and luteal phases. In the follicular phase, estradiol concentrations increase and a pituitary LH surge results in ovulation. In the luteal phase, the corpus luteum is formed with increasing progesterone secretion. If fertilization does not occur, the corpus luteum involutes. If fertilization does occur, the fetoplacental unit begins secreting β-hCG, which would help to maintain the hormonal environment of the corpus luteum.

The major sex steroids in the female are estradiol and progesterone. Much of the androgen in women originates in the ovaries, and the rest comes from the adrenal cortex and other minor sources. Androgens are primarily made in the theca cells, whereas estrogens are produced by the granulosa cells (the two-cell concept of ovarian steroidogenesis).

The embryonic gonads are indistinguishable until about six weeks. If a Y chromosome is present, the embryonic gonads become the testis. If there is no Y chromosome, the gonad becomes an ovary. The same occurs with the internal structures and external genitalia. If a testis is present, internal male structures and external male genitalia develop. In the absence of a testis, female internal structures and female external genitalia develop.

Puberty is a complex process that involves the hypothalamic-pituitary axis. All the mechanisms necessary for going into puberty are present at birth, but are held in check by stringent inhibitory mechanisms. Girls tend to start puberty earlier than boys. Ninety-nine percent of girls and boys begin going through puberty by ages 13 and 14, respectively. The adrenal glands also secrete testosterone and are important in puberty; this hormonal event is called adrenarche.

Most of the time, delayed puberty is not pathological and is simply a variation of normal (constitutional delay of puberty). X-rays of the wrist can be compared with normal standards to assess skeletal maturation. This is called a bone age study and is useful to assess the potential for further growth. Pathological causes of delayed puberty include hypopituitarism and hypogonadism.

Precocious puberty is the opposite of delayed puberty and like the latter, is usually just a variation from normal. Pathological precocious puberty results in eventual short adult stature because of premature fusion of the epiphyseal plates.

Hypogonadism may be primary or secondary. Those who contract hypogonadism before complete skeletal maturation develop what is called hypogonadal (eunuchoidal) proportions, in which the arms and legs are disproportionately long. Hypogonadism that begins after complete skeletal maturation does not alter the skeletal proportions. Hypogonadism resulting from decreased gonadotropin levels is called hypogonadotropic hypogonadism, and is the result of primary gonadal failure. Klinefelter's syndrome is the most common cause of hypergonadotropic hypogonadism in males. Turner's syndrome is another common cause of hypergonadotropic hypogonadism that occurs in females. Hypogonadism is easily treated with testosterone and estrogen supplementation.

Amenorrhea (the absence of menses) is a common complaint in women. Females with primary amenorrhea have never had a menstrual period; those with secondary amenorrhea have had menses previously but they have stopped. The most common cause of primary amenorrhea is Turner's syndrome, while the most common cause of secondary amenorrhea is anovulation.

Amenorrhea may be evaluated by administration of hormones. Administration of a progesterone derivative results in menses in women with adequate estrogenization (e.g., those with anovulation). If menses occur after administration of estrogen and progestin, this suggests a condition in which adequate estrogenization is not present (e.g., ovarian failure). If there is no bleeding with the estrogen and progestin, this suggests either the absence of the uterus or mechanical outflow obstruction.

Estrogen deficiency occurs in all women (menopause) and has many deleterious effects. Women with estrogen deficiency are at higher risk for osteoporosis. Estrogen also has beneficial cardiovascular effects, and supplementation in menopausal women helps lessen cardiovascular risk.

Polycystic ovary syndrome is a common disorder of anovulation associated with hirsutism (increased facial hair), insulin resistance, and infertility. These patients are frequently obese, and are at higher risk for developing type 2 diabetes in the future. Insulin resistance and hyperandrogenism appear to be interrelated, with each affecting the other.

LIPIDS

Lipids, or fats, provide several essential functions to the body. A primary task is providing a storage depot of energy. They place a great deal of energy into a small package (9 kcal/g, as opposed to only 4 kcal/g for carbohydrate). Triglycerides (three fatty acids esterified to a glycerol molecule) are the main storage fuel and are denser and more anhydrous than glycogen, thereby occupying less space. Some birds are able to travel thousands of miles at a time because of extremely large and calorie-dense fat stores. If the average non-obese adult has approximately 25 to 35 pounds of fat, at a caloric density of 9 kcal/g, this results in approximately 100,000

to 150,000 kcal of total body stores. At an average expenditure of 2000 kcal/day, this would last 50–75 days.

In addition, lipids are important structural parts of cell membranes (i.e., phospholipids). Cholesterol is not a fuel, but is necessary for synthesis of steroid hormones and in triglyceride metabolism. Bile acids, derived from cholesterol, act as detergents and help make nonpolar molecules soluble.

Although not a classical endocrine system, lipid metabolism is closely integrated with endocrine disorders and is thus often relegated to the endocrinologist for management.

LIPOPROTEINS

Lipids are organic molecules that are typically hydrophobic (meaning that they do not mix well with water). By themselves, they do not travel well in the bloodstream, so they require some type of carrier protein (just like many hormones do). Lipoproteins are carrier proteins that transport these hydrophobic lipid molecules in the plasma. They consist of a nonpolar lipid (triglycerides and cholesterol esters) core with an outer shell of more polar molecules (cholesterol, phospholipids, and apolipoproteins).

The four major lipoproteins in humans include chylomicrons, very low-density lipoproteins (VLDL), low-density lipoproteins (LDL), and high-density lipoproteins (HDL).

Chylomicrons are very, very large compared to the other proteins (kind of like Jupiter in our solar system) but are also the least dense, consisting mainly of triglycerides (90%), and therefore very energy rich. They transport dietary triglyceride from the gut into the lymphatics. They float to the top of plasma, forming a whitish "cream" layer. Triglycerides are removed from the chylomicrons by the enzyme lipoprotein lipase, which yields triglyceride plus chylomicron remnants. Deficiency in lipoprotein lipase results in severe hypertriglyceridemia.

LIPOPROTEIN ELECTROPHORESIS

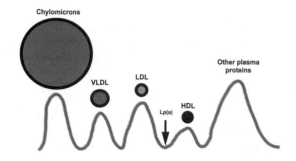

VLDL lipoproteins are next in size and consist chiefly of triglycerides, although they have less triglyceride than chylomicrons. They are important in the endogenous triglyceride pathway, transporting triglycerides made in the liver. As with chylomicrons, lipoprotein lipase removes triglyceride from VLDL, resulting in triglyceride plus IDL (intermediate-density lipoprotein).

LDL (also called β-lipoproteins) are cholesterol-rich and are a result of the degradation of VLDL. As opposed to chylomicrons and VLDL, which transport triglycerides to lymphatics for energy, LDL transport cholesterol to peripheral tissues. They are much smaller than VLDL and chylomicrons. They are taken up by LDL receptors. Increased LDL cholesterol is associated with premature atherosclerosis.

HDL (also called α-lipoproteins) are smallest in size and contain only 20% cholesterol, the rest being phospholipid and apolipoproteins. They are the densest lipoproteins and are important in removing excess cholesterol from peripheral tissues. Increased levels are associated with a decreased incidence of atherosclerosis; decreased levels correlate with increased atherosclerosis. Some people have an inherited deficiency of HDL, making them much more prone to atherosclerotic events.

Apolipoproteins are small protein components that are part of the lipoprotein structure. Some act as ligands (binding sites) for receptors, while others act as enzyme cofactors. Others provide structural integrity to the lipoprotein. Five classes exist in humans: A, B, C, D, and E.

The apo-A class of apolipoproteins is a major component of HDL, and to a lesser degree, chylomicrons and VLDL. The apo-B class is found in all lipoproteins except HDL. The major protein is apo B-100, which is the ligand for LDL to its receptor. Excess of B-100-containing lipoproteins such as LDL is bad because these molecules are atherogenic. HDL, which does not contain apo-B, is antiatherogenic.

The apo-C apolipoproteins are primary components of VLDL and chylomicrons. Apo-D is found only in HDL, and helps transfer cholesterol from HDL to apo-B rich lipoproteins (e.g., LDL) in exchange for triglyceride. The cholesterol is then taken to the liver where it is disposed. The apo-E lipoproteins are receptor ligands for VLDL, chylomicron remnants, and IDL.

Lipoprotein(a) or Lp(a) is a unique lipoprotein comprised of LDL (low-density lipoprotein) attached to a protein, apoprotein(a). Lp(a) appears to inhibit thrombus (clot) dissolution and is atherogenic. High levels are clearly linked to premature atherosclerotic disease. Those with increased Lp(a) often respond poorly to drug therapy.

HOW THE BODY OBTAINS LIPIDS

Triglycerides and cholesterol may be obtained either from diet (the exogenous lipid pathway) or degradation of lipid-rich lipoproteins (the endogenous lipid pathway). In addition, the body can synthesize cholesterol.

In the exogenous lipid pathway, dietary cholesterol is absorbed by the intestine and is incorporated into chylomicrons (which are made chiefly of triglyceride). Chylomicrons go into the lymphatic system and then the bloodstream, where the enzyme lipoprotein lipase breaks the chylomicron into triglyceride and a chylomicron remnant, which contains cholesterol ester. The liver next assimilates the chylomicron remnant where free cholesterol is isolated.

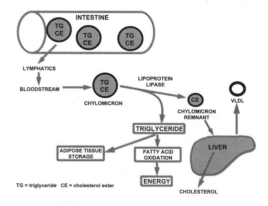

In the endogenous pathway, triglyceride- and cholesterol-rich VLDL is secreted by the liver, which is converted to triglyceride and intermediate-density lipoprotein (IDL) again by lipoprotein lipase. HDL is also involved in this process. IDL is then converted to LDL, which is taken up by tissues with an LDL receptor.

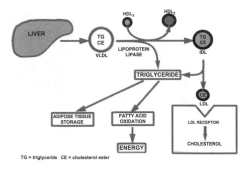

TG = triglyceride   CE = cholesterol ester

Cholesterol may also be made from acetate via a complex series of reactions. The most important step is the conversion of HMG-CoA to mevalonate by the enzyme HMG-CoA reductase. Increased cholesterol levels result in feedback inhibition of HMG-CoA reductase, thus decreasing synthesis.

HDL cholesterol is important in the reverse cholesterol pathway. Small, primordial HDL particles (nascent HDL) are secreted by the liver and intestines. Apolipoproteins bind to this immature HDL, and free cholesterol is acquired from cells, forming a slightly more advanced, small, cholesterol-poor, spherical HDL (HDL_3). Cholesterol is then attached to this HDL molecule by the enzyme LCAT (lecithin-cholesterol acyltransferase). The cholesterol molecules become more nonpolar, resulting to migration to the core and enlargement of the particle. This, along with transfer of apolipoprotein, cholesterol, and phospholipid from the delipidation of VLDL, results in a "mature" HDL particle (HDL_2). The excess cholesterol is subsequently transferred to the apo-B rich lipoproteins (LDL, VLDL, IDL, and chylomicron remnants), where they dispose of cholesterol in the liver, with excretion of the excess cholesterol as bile salts. Patients with low HDL levels therefore have decreased cholesterol removal and have an increased risk of atherosclerosis.

REVERSE CHOLESTEROL PATHWAY

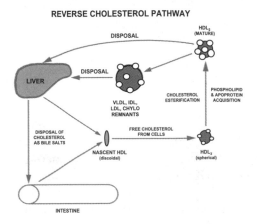

PRIMARY VERSUS SECONDARY DYSLIPIDEMIAS

Primary disorders are inherited, either as a specific gene mutation (e.g., primary hypercholesterolemia), or a polygenic disorder (e.g., familial combined hyperlipidemia).

Primary hyperlipidemias traditionally were categorized according to something called the Fredrickson classification, which characterizes lipid disorders according to the appearance (phenotype) of serum in a test tube after centrifugation. This method still carries some usefulness in the classification of primary lipid disorders and it is useful to learn at least some of the various phenotypes.

Although it seems intimidating, you can master the Fredrickson classification if you learn how lipoproteins look in serum. Chylomicrons are the least dense lipoproteins and always float to the top of plasma. Since they contain lots of hydrophobic molecules (mostly triglyceride), they have a very milky, turbid appearance. VLDL are denser than chylomicrons, and mixed with the bottom layer they do not float to the top. Since VLDL contain a large number of triglycerides, they are also somewhat turbid. HDL and LDL are clear and are virtually indistinguishable from normal plasma.

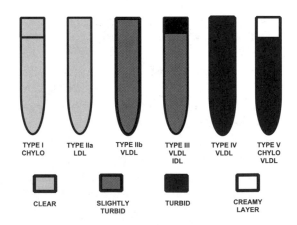

Secondary dyslipidemias are caused by diseases interfering with lipoprotein metabolism, and may also be classified according to the Fredrickson subtypes. Some secondary hyperlipidemias are more common than their primary counterparts. A common secondary disorder is type IV hyperlipidemia associated with insulin resistance and type 2 diabetes. Hypothyroidism is also very common and may result in significant LDL elevation (type IIa).

The most common primary dyslipidemia is familial combined hyperlipidemia (type IIb) and occurs in about 1 in 300 persons. It is typically manifested as moderate elevations of both triglyceride (VLDL) and LDL cholesterol. Incidence of atherogenesis is increased. It also may occur as a secondary dyslipidemia (frequently with diabetes).

Familial hypercholesterolemia (Fredrickson phenotype IIa) is another common dyslipidemia. The heterozygous (one gene present) state is most common (1 in 500), resulting in elevated LDL and typical onset of coronary artery disease between ages 40 and 50. The homozygous (both genes present) state occurs in 1 per 1,000,000 patients. LDL levels are grossly elevated and coronary disease often begins between ages 10 and 20. It is caused by a defect in the LDL receptor, resulting in increased LDL and atherosclerosis. The most common secondary cause of type IIa is hypothyroidism.

Drug therapy may be very effective for those with heterozygous type IIa disease. Homozygotes respond poorly to drug therapy, since there are few LDL receptors. Liver transplantation provides functional LDL receptors and offers the best hope in these individuals.

Familial hypertriglyceridemia (type IV hyperlipidemia), is also is a common disorder affecting approximately 1% of the population. This is a disorder of increased VLDL resulting in moderate to severe hypertriglyceridemia. The most common secondary cause of type IV is type 2 diabetes mellitus. Insulin plays a role in triglyceride removal, and impaired insulin action results in decreased clearance and hypertriglyceridemia.

Chylomicronemia syndrome or type V hyperlipidemia results from the increased accumulation of both VLDL and chylomicrons, resulting in severe hypertriglyceridemia. It is unusual as a primary lipid disorder and is usually associated with a secondary cause (such as type 2 diabetes).

Lipoprotein phenotypes may shift from one to another. For example, persons with poorly controlled diabetes often shift from type IV to V and back again after the diabetes is controlled.

PHYSICAL FINDINGS IN HYPERLIPIDEMIA

Many physical findings are present in patients with hyperlipidemia. Cholesterol accumulations called tendon xanthomas (areas of tendon thickening) may be seen in the extensor tendons (e.g., hand, patellar, and Achilles areas) in those with severe hypercholesterolemia. **They sometimes go away after cholesterol levels have been normalized.** Eruptive xanthomas are seen in severe hypertriglyceridemia. These occur on the buttocks and over extensor surfaces of the arms and legs. They are pustular lesions that wax and wane with hypertriglyceridemia.

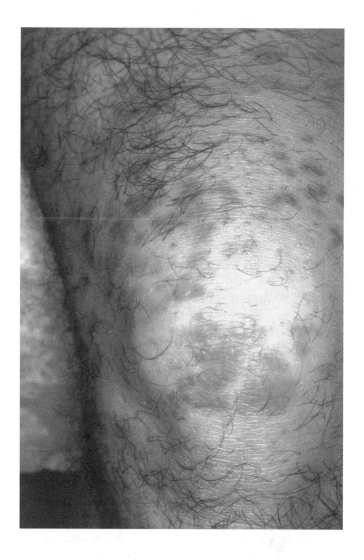

Corneal arcus is a whitish band on the outer cornea of the eye near the limbus. It is normal in elderly individuals but may indicate hypercholesterolemia in younger patients.

Xanthelasma are yellowish plaques seen near the eyelids. They are commonly seen in hypercholesterolemia but are nonspecific, as many with this finding have no lipid disorder.

Lipemia retinalis is seen in those with severe hypertriglyceridemia (usually 3000 mg/dL or greater). It is a whitish discoloration of the retinal vessels due to lipemic blood.

CONSEQUENCES OF HYPERLIPIDEMIA

Like diabetes, coronary artery disease is a major source of mortality and expense to the health care system. LDL cholesterol elevation in particular leads to increased risk of atherosclerosis. Elevations in HDL cholesterol actually protect against atherosclerosis. VLDL cholesterol elevation is usually associated with hypertriglyceridemia.

Severe hypertriglyceridemia may cause acute pancreatitis, with nausea, vomiting, and abdominal pain. Repeated attacks may result in chronic pancreatitis, pancreatic insufficiency, and even death. The significance of mild hypertriglyceridemia is less clear. In the past, it was felt that isolated hypertriglyceridemia was not a risk factor for cardiovascular disease. Hypertriglyceridemia does lower HDL levels, however, thus potentiating cardiac risk in this fashion. It is now recognized that persons with hypertriglyceridemia develop a denser, more atherogenic form of LDL—normalization of triglycerides decreases its concentration. It is now recommended that triglyceride levels be normalized, if possible, through diet or medication.

THERAPY OF HYPERLIPIDEMIA

Therapy should never be initiated based on an isolated cholesterol level. A lipoprotein profile should be obtained to identify specific abnormalities. Cholesterol may be elevated because of elevated LDL, VLDL, or even HDL. For example, LDL elevation may be treated with one type of drug, while those with VLDL cholesterol elevation might require another type of drug.

Diet is a cornerstone of therapy that unfortunately may be quite difficult for the patient. Many who are willing to take a lipid-lowering medication are unwilling to make dietary modifications. Consultation with a registered dietitian is recommended to help meal planning; and this service should be provided at a hospital or lipid clinic. It is especially important since many patients with hyperlipidemia also have diabetes.

If dietary therapy fails, lipid-lowering medication should be used. The most commonly used drugs are the reductase inhibitors (often called "statins"). These drugs are derived from fungal fermentation products and are competitive inhibitors of HMG-CoA reductase, the rate-limiting step in cholesterol biosynthesis. They are extremely effective at reducing LDL cholesterol, are easily taken, and well tolerated. They are less useful for the treatment of hypertriglyceridemia. Examples include lovastatin, atorvastatin, and simvastatin. These drugs rarely cause myositis and hepatic transaminase elevation.

Fibric acid derivatives (fibrates) are primarily used in the treatment of hypertriglyceridemia. They are less effective than statins for isolated LDL elevation. Fibrates work by increasing VLDL and chylomicron clearance, and inhibiting VLDL production. Examples include gemfibrozil and fenofibrate.

Resins or bile acid sequestrants are charged molecules that bind bile acids in the intestine. Since much of the body's cholesterol is derived from the recirculating "pool" of bile acids, diminishing the size of the pool decreases the body's cholesterol. This bile acid-resin complex is then eliminated in the stool. Common side effects of resins include constipation and bloating. Resins should be taken alone, since they are highly charged molecules, and may bind and impair the absorption of other medications. For poorly understood reasons, resins may increase VLDL synthesis and therefore exacerbate preexisting hypertriglyceridemia, and should be avoided in patients with triglyceride problems. Available resins include cholestyramine and colestipol. These are the only lipid-lowering medications that are not systemically absorbed by the body.

Nicotinic acid (niacin, vitamin B-3) is required for normal metabolism but has potent lipid-lowering characteristics in large doses. (It is not related to nicotine, a toxic alkaloid found in tobacco and pesticides.) Niacin has been used for many years and is an excellent treatment for both LDL cholesterol elevation and hypertriglyceridemia. Modest HDL cholesterol elevation also occurs.

Niacin is the Dr. Jekyll and Mr. Hyde of lipid lowering medications. The Dr. Jekyll–form helps lower LDL and triglyceride levels. The Mr. Hyde–side of niacin is seen in its many side effects. The most frequent is cutaneous flushing, similar to the menopausal hot flash. This reaction is caused by prostaglandins and often averted by giving inhibitors of prostaglandin synthesis (e.g., aspirin).

Niacin may raise blood glucose and must be used with caution in individuals with impaired glucose tolerance or diabetes mellitus. Unfortunately, these individuals are often the ones with severe hypertriglyceridemia that require niacin therapy—a tough situation. One advantage of niacin is its low cost.

Omega-3 fatty acids are contained in marine (fish) oils and significantly lower VLDL cholesterol (and therefore triglyceride) levels in hyperlipidemic patients. Little or no change occurs in those with normal lipids or with isolated cholesterol elevation. They also appear to have anti-atherogenic effects that are independent of the lipid-lowering effects, possibly due to their effect on prostaglandin metabolism. They may be of use in patients with severe hypertriglyceridemia unresponsive to fibrates and/or niacin. They increase hepatic glucose production and must be used with caution in those with diabetes. They also make the patient smell like fish!

Probucol is an antioxidant that causes modest LDL cholesterol reduction, via increased clearance. Unfortunately, this drug also reduces HDL cholesterol. Although in theory antioxidants may prevent atherogenesis, this has not been demonstrated in clinical studies. Probucol is only rarely used and is not a good first-line agent for hyperlipidemia.

DISORDERS OF MULTIPLE ENDOCRINE GLANDS AND PARANEOPLASTIC SYNDROMES

REVIEW

Let's review what we learned in the last lecture. Lipids provide several essential functions to the body. Their most important function is to provide long-term energy storage. Lipids are also important as precursors for hormones and structural components of cell membranes.

There are four major lipoproteins in humans. These include chylomicrons, very low-density lipoproteins (VLDL), low-density lipoproteins (LDL), and high-density lipoproteins (HDL). Chylomicrons are the least dense and float to the top of plasma if left standing in a test tube; they consist chiefly of triglycerides. VLDL lipoproteins are also very triglyceride-rich and carry cholesterol as well. LDL is very cholesterol-rich and is an important factor in atherogenesis. HDL is the smallest lipoprotein and is important in removing cholesterol from peripheral tissues. Increased HDL is thus inversely correlated with atherosclerosis. Apolipoproteins are the building blocks of lipoproteins.

There are several important pathways of lipid metabolism in humans. The endogenous lipid pathway is how the body obtains lipids from the diet. In this system, triglyceride-rich chylomicrons are absorbed by the lymphatic system. Cholesterol is later isolated from chylomicron remnants by the liver. In the endogenous pathway, the liver secretes triglyceride and cholesterol-rich VLDL particles, which are then converted to free triglyceride and other particles by lipoprotein lipase. LDL is formed, which is taken up by tissues with an LDL receptor.

In addition, the body may make its own cholesterol. The rate-limiting step of cholesterol biosynthesis is catalyzed by the enzyme HMG-CoA reductase.

Lipoprotein disorders may be classified as primary or secondary. Primary lipid disorders are inherited. Secondary disorders are caused by another disorder, such as diabetes. Both types of lipid disorders are sometimes classified according to the Fredrickson scheme, which groups lipid phenotypes according to the appearance of serum in a test tube.

The most common primary dyslipidemia is familial combined (type IIb) hyperlipidemia. The second most common is familial hypercholesterolemia (type IIa). Those with heterozygous type IIa disease often develop premature atherosclerosis by the ages of 40 to 50. Those with homozygous disease may develop disease in the second or third decades of life. Other types of primary hyperlipidemia are uncommon.

Diabetes is a common cause of secondary hyperlipidemia, frequently resulting in type IV and type V hyperlipidemia. Hypothyroidism frequently results in type IIa hyperlipidemia.

Multiple clinical studies have demonstrated decreased morbidity and mortality from coronary artery disease in aggressive therapy of patients with hyperlipidemia. Atherosclerosis is most commonly linked to elevated LDL cholesterol, although hypertriglyceridemia has also been shown to play a role in atherosclerosis. Many patients with hypertriglyceridemia also have diabetes.

The first line of treatment in hyperlipidemia is diet therapy, which may be difficult for some patients. Multiple pharmacologic agents are also available. The most useful are the HMG-CoA reductase inhibitors (statins), which inhibit cholesterol synthesis and result in dramatic lowering of LDL cholesterol. Fibric acid derivatives (fibrates) are useful in treatment of hypertriglyceridemia. Nicotinic acid (niacin) is a useful drug in the treatment of both hypercholesterolemia and hypertriglyceridemia, but use is limited by its frequent unpleasant side effects. Resins or bile acid sequestrants are useful in patients with mild to moderate LDL cholesterol elevations.

POLYENDOCRINE SYNDROMES

We have thus far discussed endocrine disorders specific to the organ system. This lecture attempts to "put it all together" and discuss disorders that affect more than one endocrine system—the polyendocrine disorders. Lastly, I will discuss the so-called ectopic endocrine or paraneoplastic syndromes—endocrine disorders resulting from secretion of hormones from non-endocrine-system tumors.

These disorders involve more than one endocrine system and may be divided into (a) the immunoendocrine syndromes and (b) the multiple endocrine neoplasia (MEN) syndromes. With few exceptions, the former are disorders of endocrine deficiency while the latter are syndromes of endocrine excess. They are typically confused with one another, although they are fundamentally different disorders.

The immunoendocrine disorders are autoimmune syndromes that affect multiple endocrine organs. The first was described in 1926 by Schmidt, who reported autopsy findings in two patients with "a two-gland illness" (adrenal insufficiency and hypothyroidism). This syndrome may also be associated with other disorders and is sometimes called Schmidt's syndrome, or polyglandular autoimmune syndrome type II (PGA II). It is important to be aware of these syndromes, since a patient with one autoimmune endocrine disorder may be at risk for developing further endocrine disorders. They are genetically transmitted and so genetic counseling and surveillance of family members is important.

Type II polyglandular syndrome (Schmidt's syndrome) is the most common of the endocrine deficiency syndromes. It involves the occurrence of two or more of the following autoimmune endocrine disorders in the same individual: Addison's disease, Hashimoto's thyroiditis, Graves' disease, type 1 diabetes mellitus, and/or primary gonadal failure. Note that Graves' disease is unique because it is an autoimmune disorder of hormonal excess; the others are deficiency syndromes. Pernicious anemia and vitiligo also may be seen.

In order to qualify, the disorders must be autoimmune; i.e., adrenal failure due to histoplasmosis, hypothyroidism due to thyroidectomy, and type 2 diabetes do not count.

The individual diseases are identical to—and are treated just like—those that occur individually. One disease may commonly exacerbate another, however (e.g., adrenal insufficiency aggravates hypoglycemic responsiveness in type 1 diabetics and hyperthyroidism aggravates adrenal insufficiency).

The type I syndrome is much less common and primarily seen in children. It is usually associated with Addison's disease, mucocutaneous candidiasis, and hypoparathyroidism. Other endocrine abnormalities are rarely seen (much less commonly than in PGA II) and include hypothyroidism, Graves' disease, gonadal failure, and diabetes mellitus.

MULTIPLE ENDOCRINE NEOPLASIA (MEN)

Multiple endocrine neoplasia (MEN) syndromes are associated with multiple endocrine tumors, benign and malignant, which result in syndromes of hormone excess. Hormone deficiency may occasionally occur as the result of destructive effects of a large tumor (e.g., pituitary). MEN syndromes are divided into two broad categories: MEN I and MEN IIa/IIb.

MEN I is characterized by the "three Ps"—pituitary, pancreatic islet, and parathyroid tumors. Two or more tumors in the same individual are diagnostic for MEN. Hyperparathyroidism is the most common manifestation, occurring in over 95% of those affected. By age 40, almost all carrying the gene have hypercalcemia. Pancreatic islet cell tumors are the second most common manifestation, occurring in up to 80% of patients. The tumors are typically multicentric and therefore surgical cure is difficult. Pharmacologic treatment of the hormone excess is often required.

The most common pancreatic tumor is a gastrinoma, leading to Zollinger-Ellison syndrome (gastric acid hypersecretion), multiple peptic ulcers, and diarrhea. Serum gastrin levels are usually elevated. Treatment includes histamine-2 (H_2) antagonists (e.g., cimetidine, ranitidine) and/or proton pump inhibitors (omeprazole), and gastrectomy may be required. Since the pancreatic peptide somatostatin inhibits gastrin secretion, the long-acting somatostatin analog octreotide may be useful.

Insulinoma is the second most common islet cell tumor. This results in severe fasting hypoglycemia with inappropriately elevated serum insulin and C-peptide concentrations. Seizures and death may occur if untreated. As these tumors are usually multicentric, total pancreatectomy may be required.

Pituitary adenomas are the third most common manifestation and occur in over 50% of patients with MEN I. These include prolactin, growth hormone, and ACTH-secreting tumors, with the associated clinical manifestations. Tumors may also be nonfunctional and cause compressive symptoms if large enough.

Carcinoid tumors also may occur but are the least common tumor type. These produce large amounts of serotonin and cause severe flushing and diarrhea. Lipomas (subcutaneous and visceral) are also associated, but do not produce hormones.

MEN IIa is the association of medullary thyroid carcinoma with pheochromocytoma and, less commonly, hyperparathyroidism. Calcitonin levels are usually elevated in these patients. Pheochromocytoma presents with the typical manifestations of hypertension, tachycardia, headaches, hyperhidrosis, and cardiac arrhythmias. Clinical history and elevation of serum or urine catecholamines and metabolites typically establish the diagnosis. MRI or CT may localize the tumor. Hyperparathyroidism may also be present, although much less commonly than in MEN I (10–20% of MEN IIa as opposed to >90% of MEN I).

MEN type IIb is the combination of medullary thyroid carcinoma, pheochromocytoma, multiple mucosal neuromas, and a characteristic marfanoid habitus (long, thin body habitus with arachnodactyly). Hyperparathyroidism is not seen in this disorder.

PARANEOPLASTIC SYNDROMES

These are also called ectopic or "out of place" endocrine syndromes, since the hormones are produced by tumors of non-endocrine origin. For example, insulin produced by a pancreatic insulinoma is not a paraneoplastic syndrome since the tumor normally makes this substance. These disorders were first recognized by the association of hypercalcemia with certain malignancies. In this lecture we will discuss the most common paraneoplastic syndromes.

The most common ectopic syndrome is hypercalcemia, and is usually caused by secretion of a substance called PTH-related peptide (PTH-rP). This syndrome is termed humoral hypercalcemia of malignancy (HHM). Another type of paraneoplastic hypercalcemia is called local osteolytic hypercalcemia (LOH), and accounts for most of the remaining patients with paraneoplastic hypercalcemia. LOH is caused by osteoclast activating factors (OAFs) that cause bone destruction (lysis) and hypercalcemia. Very rarely, some hematologic malignancies (lymphomas) may produce calcitriol, resulting in a type of vitamin D-dependent hypercalcemia.

How do we distinguish humoral hypercalcemia of malignancy (HHM) from primary hyperparathyroidism? By measuring PTH-rP. In HHM, native PTH levels will be suppressed, because of normal feedback on the parathyroids, while the level of PTH-rP is elevated. In hyperparathyroidism, PTH levels are high, while PTH-rP levels are low. HHM is very aggressive, while hyperparathyroidism typically presents with mild hypercalcemia that progresses slowly over several years.

SIADH (syndrome of inappropriate antidiuretic hormone) is the next most common paraneoplastic syndrome. It is usually obvious that this is a paraneoplastic syndrome, since tumors of the native gland do not produce this condition.

Cushing's syndrome due to ectopic ACTH secretion is the third most common ectopic syndrome. Since the tumor (usually small-cell lung carcinoma) is typically quite aggressive, the clinical appearance may evolve over weeks, as compared to the relatively indolent Cushing's due to pituitary tumors, which may take months to years to notice. Cushing's syndrome due to adrenal tumors can be easily differentiated from ectopic ACTH syndrome, since ACTH levels are low in the former. If the distinction between Cushing's disease and ectopic ACTH syndrome is not obvious, petrosal sinus (blood draining the pituitary) sampling can be done. With Cushing's disease, petrosal sinus ACTH is greater than peripheral blood ACTH. The high-dose dexamethasone suppression test can also be useful, if desired. A less common type of ectopic ACTH syndrome associated with bronchial carcinoids is less aggressive, and may be harder to distinguish from Cushing's disease.

Treatment of paraneoplastic syndromes is directed at the primary tumor. If tumor shrinkage occurs, hormone secretion also diminishes and the syndrome improves. Specific antagonist therapy may be required in conjunction with antitumor therapy.

Hypercalcemia of malignancy due to PTH-rP is best treated with inhibitors of bone resorption (pamidronate, etidronate). Calcitonin is a weak antagonist and is useful only in mild cases. More potent but toxic antiresorptive agents include gallium nitrate and the antitumor antibiotic plicamycin (mithramycin). Patients are usually dehydrated and normal saline administration promotes calciuresis. Radiation therapy may benefit those with local osteolytic hypercalcemia (LOH). Those with hypercalcemia due to immunologic factors or calcitriol respond to glucocorticoids.

SIADH usually is treated with fluid restriction and management of the underlying disease. In refractory cases, demeclocycline, which produces ADH resistance (and thus a state of nephrogenic diabetes insipidus), may be used.

Ectopic ACTH syndrome may be treated with drugs that inhibit adrenal steroid synthesis, such as ketoconazole, aminoglutethimide, and metyrapone. The aldosterone antagonist spironolactone aids in correcting the hypokalemia. If these measures are unsuccessful, bilateral adrenalectomy may be required. These patients typically have a poor prognosis.

GLOSSARY

Acromegaly - Disorder resulting from excess growth hormone in adults.

ACTH (adrenocorticotropic hormone) - Protein hormone secreted by the anterior pituitary; results in increased glucocorticoid synthesis.

Addison's disease - Primary adrenal insufficiency, usually caused by autoimmune disease.

Aldosterone - Mineralocorticoid made in zona glomerulosa of adrenal cortex.

Amenorrhea - Condition of absent menses; may be primary (menses never occurred) or secondary (previous menses have stopped).

Anabolic - Metabolic processes that create molecules; occur in well-fed state.

Angiotensin II - Potent vasoconstrictor produced in the liver upon stimulation from renin; trophic hormone for aldosterone secretion.

Antidiuretic hormone (ADH, vasopressin) - Posterior pituitary hormone important in water metabolism.

Apolipoproteins - Subcomponents of lipoprotein molecules; various types exist.

Autoimmune disease - Disorders caused by antibodies produced by the body against its own organs.

Becquerel - Unit of radionuclide activity; 1 Ci (curie) = 37 GBq (gigabecquerels).

Beta (β) particle - Electron emitted from an atom's nucleus after decay; negatively charged.

Bile acid sequestrants (resins) - Drugs which bind cholesterol in the intestine and prevent its recirculation; useful in hypercholesterolemia.

Calcitonin - Protein hormone made by the parafollicular cells of the thyroid; regulator of calcium metabolism.

Catabolic - Metabolic processes that break down molecules for fuel; useful when organism needs food.

Catecholamines - Hormones derived from tyrosine and secreted by adrenal medulla and other neural tissues, e.g., norepinephrine, epinephrine.

Cholesterol - A molecule that plays an important role in atherosclerosis and also serves as a precursor of steroid and sterol hormones.

Chylomicrons - Large, buoyant lipoproteins important in carrying dietary triglyceride to cells.

Colloid - Proteinacious substance in the thyroid follicle containing thyroglobulin and iodothyronine molecules.

Computed tomography (CT) - Uses conventional x-ray beams to produce high-resolution "cross-sections" of a body part.

Congenital adrenal hyperplasia - Disorder of adrenal enzyme synthesis resulting in accumulation of steroid precursors, with varying deleterious effects.

Cortisol (hydocortisone) - Glucocorticoid made in zona fasciculata of adrenal cortex.

Cortisone - Derivative of cortisol.

CRH (corticotropin-releasing hormone) - Hypothalamic hormone that stimulates ACTH secretion.

Curie - Unit of radionuclide activity; 1 Ci = 3.7×10^{10} disintegrations per second.

Cushing's disease - Type of Cushing's syndrome caused by an ACTH-secreting pituitary tumor.

Cushing's syndrome - Disorder resulting from excess glucocorticoids.

Cytokines - Mediators secreted by immune cells; important in regulation of many endocrine processes.

Diabetes insipidus - Disorder of excessive thirst and urination resulting from inadequate antidiuretic hormone.

Diabetes mellitus - Disorder of ineffective glucose metabolism.

Dopamine - Catecholamine hormone produced by adrenal medulla and other neuroendocrine tissue; inhibits prolactin and TSH secretion.

Endogenous - Originates from inside the body, e.g., endogenous hyperthyroidism.

Epinephrine - Catecholamine hormone produced by adrenal medulla and other neuroendocrine tissue.

Estradiol - Primary estrogen (female hormone); secreted by ovary.

Euthyroid sick syndrome - Condition in which alterations in protein binding lead to low total T3 and/or T4 levels with normal free levels in euthyroid patients.

Exogenous - Originates from outside the body, e.g., exogenous corticosteroid ingestion.

Feedback inhibition - Regulatory mechanism; increase or decrease in hormone levels result in appropriate degree of stimulation by trophic hormone.

Fibric acid derivatives - Drugs useful in treatment of hypertriglyceridemia.

Fludrocortisone - Synthetic mineralocorticoid used in treatment of adrenal insufficiency.

FSH (follicle-stimulating hormone) - A glycoprotein hormone made by the anterior pituitary gland, important in gonadal regulation.

Gamma rays - High-energy photons emitted from an atom's nucleus after a nuclear event (e.g., ejection of an electron).

GHRH (growth hormone-releasing hormone) - Hypothalamic hormone that stimulates GH secretion.

Gigantism - Disorder resulting from excess growth hormone in children.

Glucagon - Protein hormone made by pancreatic alpha cells; antagonist to insulin.

Glycogen - Short-term fuel comprised of multiple glucose molecules; stored in liver and muscle.

Glycoprotein - A protein molecule attached to sugars.

GnRH (gonadotropin hormone-releasing hormone) - Hypothalamic hormone that stimulates LH and FSH secretion.

Goiter - Enlargement of the thyroid; may be nodular or diffuse.

Graves' disease - Common cause of hyperthyroidism caused by antibodies which mimic TSH action on the thyroid.

Growth hormone (GH) - Anterior pituitary hormone important in normal growth and development.

Gynecomastia - Abnormal breast tissue development in males; usually a benign condition.

Hashimoto's thyroiditis - Also called Hashimoto's disease; common endocrine disorder often resulting in goiter and hypothyroidism.

HDL (high-density lipoprotein) - Scavenger lipoprotein important in removing cholesterol from cells.

Hermaphrodite - Person containing reproductive organs of both sexes.

Hirsutism - Abnormal terminal (dark) hair growth in women.

HMG-CoA reductase - Rate-limiting enzyme in cholesterol biosynthesis; site of attack of many lipid-lowering drugs.

HMG-CoA reductase inhibitors (statins) - Potent inhibitors of cholesterol biosynthesis; useful in lowering LDL cholesterol.

Hydrocortisone - Same as cortisol.

Hyperthyroidism - Any condition resulting in increased thyroid hormone levels.

Hypoglycemia - Condition of decreased serum glucose, resulting in symptoms of hypoglycemia; symptoms resolve after treatment.

Hypogonadism - Condition resulting from decreased sex steroids.

Hypoparathyroidism - Condition of parathyroid hormone deficiency, resulting in hypocalcemia and hypophosphatemia.

Hypothyroidism - Condition where too little thyroid hormone exists.

Insulin - Protein hormone made by pancreatic beta cells; important in normal glucose metabolism.

Iodothyronines - Thyroid hormones, e.g., T4 (thyroxine) and T3 (triiodothyronine).

Kallmann's syndrome - Syndrome of hypogonadotropic hypogonadism resulting from defect in GnRH secretion.

Klinefelter's syndrome - Common cause of hypergonadotropic hypogonadism in males, resulting from 47, XXY chromosomal defect.

LDL (low-density lipoprotein) - Atherogenic lipoprotein that carries cholesterol to cells.

Leydig cells - Testicular cells which are the site of testosterone production.

LH (luteinizing hormone) - A glycoprotein hormone made by the anterior pituitary gland, important in gonadal regulation.

Lipids - Molecues that provide long-term energy for the body (triglycerides) and other functions; some are atherogenic.

Lipoprotein - Molecule that carries lipids throughout the body.

Magnetic resonance imaging (MRI) - Uses high-powered magnetic fields to produce images based on oscillation of hydrogen nuclei.

Metformin - Oral diabetes drug that decreases hepatic glucose output and improves insulin sensitivity in type 2 diabetics.

Multinodular goiter - Thyroid gland with two or more nodules; may be euthyroid or toxic.

Nicotinic acid (niacin) - Vitamin B-3; useful drug for hyperlipidemia in high doses.

Norepinephrine - Catecholamine hormone produced by adrenal medulla and other neuroendocrine tissue.

Nuclear medicine - Science in which radioactive substances given to patients may be used for imaging or therapy.

Osteomalacia - Condition caused by decreased calcium formation in bone.

Osteoporosis - Disorder of decreased bone mass.

Panhypopituitarism - Deficiency of all pituitary hormones.

Paraneoplastic (ectopic) syndrome - Endocrine disorder resulting from secretion of a hormone by cell type not normally associated with it.

Parathyroid hormone - Protein hormone manufactured by parathyroid glands; important regulator of calcium metabolism.

Parathyroid hormone-related protein - PTH-like protein important in fetal development; may cause hypercalcemia if secreted by certain malignancies.

Polycystic ovary syndrome - Disorder of chronic anovulation resulting in amenorrhea, infertility, and hyperandrogenism.

Positron - β particle with a positive charge.

Precocious puberty - Condition in which puberty commences too early; may be complete (central or true), or incomplete (peripheral).

PRH (prolactin-releasing hormone) - Hypothalamic hormone that increases pituitary prolactin production; recently isolated.

Primary endocrine disorder - Defect lies in the target gland itself.

Progesterone - Steroid hormone important in female reproductive cycle.

Prolactin - Anterior pituitary hormone important in mammalian lactation.

Prostaglandins - Hormones formed from fatty acids; play a variety of biological roles.

Protein - A molecule, often large, comprised of many amino acids.

Pseudohermaphrodite - Person whose phenotype (appearance) is opposite that of the genetic sex.

Pseudohypoparathyroidism - Disorder of parathyroid hormone resistance; often occurs with characteristic physical anomalies.

Radioactive iodine - Typically ^{123}I or ^{131}I; usually used as sodium iodide (NaI) in thyroid imaging or treatment.

Meglinitides - Drugs (e.g., repaglinidie, natiglinide) which enhance insulin production by pancreas; useful as oral agent for diabetes.

Rickets - Consequence of vitamin D deficiency in children.

Second messenger - Produced by hormones that bind to cell surface receptors; have biologic effect on nucleus.

Secondary endocrine disorder - Defect lies in the secretion of the trophic hormone for the target gland.

Secretagogue - Substance used in perturbation tests of endocrine function that stimulates hormone secretion.

Sertoli cells - Testicular cells which are the site of sperm production.

SIADH (syndrome of inappropriate antidiuretic hormone secretion) - Condition of ADH excess resulting in retention of free water and hyponatremia.

Somatostatin - Hormone produced by hypothalamus and pancreas; inhibitory effects on several hormones.

Spironolactone - Androgen and aldosterone antagonist useful in treating hyperaldosteronism and hirsutism.

StAR (steroidogenic acute regulatory protein) - Important in transferring cholesterol to mitochondria for corticosteroid synthesis.

Sulfonylureas - Oral hypoglycemic agent that increased endogenous insulin secretion.

Syndrome X - Syndrome of hyperinsulinemia, hypertension, glucose intolerance, hyperlipidemia, and atherosclerosis.

T3 resin uptake - Indirect measurement of thyroid binding proteins; correlates inversely with protein levels.

Technetium - Man-made radioactive element important in nuclear medicine.

Tertiary endocrine disorder - Defect lies one step higher than the trophic hormone (e.g., hypothalamic dysfunction).

Testicular feminization - Syndrome of androgen resistance resulting in normal female phenotype in a genetic male.

Testosterone - Primary androgen (male hormone); secreted by testis and adrenal gland.

Thiazolidinediones - Insulin-sensitizing drugs useful in the treatment of type 2 diabetes.

Thyroglobulin - Protein upon which thyroid hormones are synthesized and stored in the thyroid follicle.

Thyroid-binding globulin (TBG) - Major thyroid hormone transport protein.

Thyrotoxicosis - Condition in which excess thyroid hormone is present in the blood; of endogenous origin.

Thyroxine (T4) - Principal hormone secreted by the thyroid gland.

TRH (thyrotropin-releasing hormone) - Hypothalamic hormone that increases pituitary TSH production.

Triglycerides - Energy-rich component of adipose tissue.

Triiodothyronine (T3) - Most active thyroid hormone; mainly formed by peripheral conversion of T4 in the blood.

Trophic hormone - Hormone that stimulates another hormone's production.

TSH (thyroid-stimulating hormone) - A glycoprotein hormone made by the anterior pituitary gland, important in thyroid regulation.

Turner's syndrome - Common cause of hypergonadotropic hypogonadism in females; typical 45X karyotype, short stature, webbed neck, and infertility.

Tyrosine - Amino acid used as building block of catecholamine and iodothyronine hormones.

Ultrasound - Imaging modality using the attenuation of high-frequency sound waves through matter.

Vitamin D - Sterol hormone important in normal calcium absorption from the intestine.

VLDL (very low-density lipoprotein) - Triglyceride-rich lipoprotein important in carrying endogenous triglyceride to cells.

X-rays - High-energy photons emitted from an atom's electron shell after a nuclear event.